YOGA ON GO

The joyous experience of a nuclear engineer turned Yoga teacher-technology & yoga can truly blend into daily life

Raghuvir (Ravi) Rustagi

YOGA-ON-GO

Wishes the readers a successful yogic journey

D0111774

PRAISE FOR YOGA ON GO

First of all I would like to congratulate you on the excellent book, with a very meticulous, and pragmatic compilation of basic principles and most useful practices.

I hope this book will also remove the most common myth (inconvenient truth of most young people) of being too busy, and pave the way for better health.

I plan to read and follow it more thoroughly myself and will share it with other family members.

Ashok K. Singhal, Ph.D.

Founder & Chairman of CFD Research Corporation

Co-Chairman for SynVivo, Inc.

Congratulations on publishing this great book. I know you have been working on this book for some time. I will defiantly recommend this book to my friends and relatives.

Jag Chopra

Prof Ravi Rustagi has been volunteering and sharing his Yoga Knowledge with many of us in the Livingston, NJ area. He has coined the phrase YOG >> Yoga On the Go! My Posture when I sit, or walk has improved dramatically. I am more aware when I am slouching! His emphasis on Rhythmic Breathing, Pranayam, and Various Asanas have helped many in our senior community.

Tarun Mehta

This is an excellent book, guiding us how to maintain and achieve perfect health in simple and practical ways. Five stars to The Author of this excellent book Prof Ravi Ji Rustagi Thanks

Daksha & Hasmukh Modi Livingston, NJ.

DISCLAIMER

The writings in this eBook are intended as information on yogic living and not a substitute for professional medical diagnosis, cure, or treatment for any ailment. The author, the Sambandh group, or the publisher of this Book disclaims all responsibility for any loss, injury, or liability, directly or indirectly, incurred due to the use or application of practices described in this Book.

Author: Raghuvir (Ravi) Rustagi

ravirustagi16@gmail.com

The eBook is divided into three parts for ease of absorption

PART ONE: What is Yoga- it is a healer; practice it

PART TWO: Why do Yoga- it is a science; experiment with it

PART THREE: How to do Yoga- practice it; make it a lifestyle

The Book explores yoga techniques to let you evolve, transform, experience, and be a better self.

TABLE OF CONTENTS

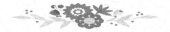

Praise for YOGA ON GO.. i

PREFACE ix

PART ONE: 1

WHAT IS YOGA?.. 1

    ACTS 1 - 12 ARE PRESENTED FOR SELF-STUDY................................ 3

    INTRO 7

    ACT-1: SIT STEADY & BE PAIN-FREE 17

    ACT- 2: PREVENT FALLS 21

    ACT- 3: WALK FATIGUE-FREE 29

    ACT- 4: BEND & LIFT SAFE 37

    ACT- 5: BREATHE BETTER 39

    ACT- 6: TECHNIQUES OF PRANAYAMA 47

    ACT- 7: BE CALM, & FOCUSED.. 55

    ACT- 8: THE POWER OF POSITIVE 61

    ACT- 9: SLEEP WELL EVERY NIGHT 65

    ACT- 10: MANAGING EMOTION CURES DEPRESSION 69

    ACT- 11: YOUR RIGHTS TO REDEEM.................................... 75

    ACT- 12: MEDITATE DAILY.. 77

    CONCLUSION: PART ONE 87

PART TWO: 89

WHY DO YOGA?.. 89

    22-TOPICS ON SWADHYAYA FOR STUDY OF SELF SVATMA............ 91

    1. WHY CHOOSE YOG PLUS GYM 93

2. FOUR GREAT QUESTIONS (MAHAVAKYAS) 95

3. SANKHYA YOG...AT A GLANCE.....................................97

4. FIVE BODIES TO THE SELF (*PANCH KOSH/LAYERS*) 101

5. ETERNAL LAWS/TRUTHS OF NATURE 105

6. YOUR SPIRITUAL METER 109

7. FOUR PILLARS (PURUSHARTHAS) 111

8. SAMSKARAS ARE FORMED 4 WAYS 115

9. MINDFULNESS VS. MEDITATION 117

10. AHAR, VIHAR, ACHAR, VICHAR - DYNAMIC LIFESTYLE 119

11. FOOD IS MEDICINE- CHALLENGE YOUR KNOWLEDGE OF DIET 121

12. SENIOR FITNESS 125

13. THREE GUNAS (DYNAMIC ATTRIBUTES OF NATURE) 127

14. SEVEN ENERGY CENTERS: CHAKRAS- 101 131

15. PURITY PRACTICE 133

16. ACCESSORIES/SUPPORTS 137

17. PATANJALI'S YOG-DARSHAN 2000-YEAR-OLD BOOK..............141

18. POPULAR YOGA PATHS & MODES OF POSTURES 145

19.1 BUILD DAILY HOME PRACTICE (20 MIN/DAY) 147

19.2 CURE FOR ANXIETY/HYPERTENSION/HIGH BP......................149

19.3 BUILD HOME PRACTICE (1-HR) FOR TOTAL HEALTH.............151

19.4 BUILD HOME PRACTICE FOR PROSTATE HEALTH..................153

19.5 HOME CARE FOR SPINE HEALTH-TWIST & BEND.................157

19.6 SELECTED ASANAS FOR YOUNG ADULTS/STUDENTS............159

20. UPASANA – PRAYER 161

21. MANTRA, PRAYER & MEANING 163

22. CONCLUSION: PART TWO 165

REFRESH THE BASICS..167

PART THREE: 171

HOW TO YOGA? 171

    1. MAKE YOG A SUBTLE, HIGHER STYLE OF HEALING 173

    2. CELEBRATING YOG 175

    3. INDIVIDUAL VS. COLLECTIVE KARMA 177

    4. YOG IS DANCE 179

    5. YOG IS FUN 181

    6. LIST OF 28 CONTRIBUTORS 183

    7. DEMO POSTURES 185

    8. MORE ASANAS FOR MINDFULNESS 203

    9. MYSTERY (MY STORY) OF HEALTH 207

    10. INSOMNIA: SAVASAN & YOG-NIDRA 209

    11. FOUR (4) PRINCIPLES OF AYURVEDA 211

    12. CONSTIPATION 213

    13. EYE CARE 215

    14. SUN SALUTATION 217

    15. SUN SALUTATION - EXPLANATION OF BENEFITS 219

    16. ASANAS ARE EXERCISES AT A SUBTLE LEVEL 221

    17. YOGA FOR HIGHER VIRTUES- SIMPLIFIED 227

    18. NOVEL WELLNESS REPORT 229

    19. NOVEL GREETING CARD DESIGN 231

    20. CONCLUSION: PART THREE 233

    ACKNOWLEDGMENTS 237

    ABOUT THE AUTHOR 239

    REFERENCES 243

PREFACE

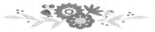

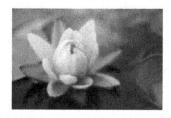

'Yoga On Go' (YOG) promotes yoga as logical and sacred but not an ascetic discipline.

- A Lotus grows in filth yet retains its untarnished glory.

- Lotus teaches: the world is not a curse, and you can be in it, not of it?

- Indian sages have described the world as a boat.

The boat merrily floats in water but does not let water become the boat.

Originated in India, Yoga is one of the oldest health practices in the world. The basic principle in yoga is the body, mind, and spirit are the three entities in every human being. If the body is sick, it affects the mind and spirit and vice versa. Yoga makes you aware that health means the three entities are **balanced** and in team spirit. For example:

- To begin, you may be a theist, atheist, or just curious.

- As the practice matures, you'd learn that human nature is inherently Divine. This upgrade in longing transforms your status from a curious onlooker to an ardent seeker.

- **Do this dynamic balancing as you go, more so at sadhana hour, by expressing gratitude to God.**

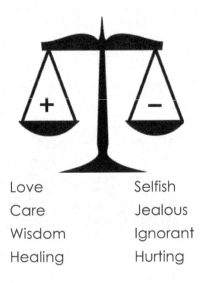

Love	Selfish
Care	Jealous
Wisdom	Ignorant
Healing	Hurting

Q: A novice may ask, which side wins +, or -?
A: The side you promote wins.

The power of choice is in your hands. The finest steel is made in the hottest furnace (Tapas)

Trees with the most magnificent branches also have the deepest roots (Tadasan)

There are advocates for the prevention of child & domestic abuse. YOG is an advocate for the prevention of self-abuse.

The challenge is to realize that your true ID is the inner Reality

Survive means an ordinary mind- content to live an easy, safe, comfortable life, mainly to fulfil the craving of bodily senses and make meaningless habits.

Thrive means a planned, trained growth thru an evolved mindset

Example 1 - A desire to eat is natural, and there is nothing wrong with it.

An ordinary mind: You choose the food to satisfy the taste buds and fill the belly. You may eat organic meat dishes and drink imported wine to wash down. Yet, you're eating expensive 'junk,' making useless habits of selfishness, fear, anger, and greed.

An evolved mind: You will additionally inquire if the food is nutritious and beneficial to the body/mind. You're now functioning higher, and self-discovery is your goal.

Example 2 – Random action, speech, and thinking come naturally to all people. The right breathing and right posture are reserved for the Yog-Conscious.

YOG, as taught in this Book: You learn how to function at any moment above and beyond the usual comfort zone. It is OK to find a few minutes in the morning and evening if a full one hour is not feasible.

YOG can be a way to take a break, close your eyes and take a look in your in-box.

Yoga On Go is a set of asanas/postures/tips for inspiring seniors, retirees, and young adults so that they can keep healthy, inhibit disease, and aid recovery from an unexpected sickness. By following a yogic lifestyle, you'll win the ongoing battle between the past and present karmas, good and not-so-good habits/samskaras in the struggles of life.

A professional engineer, now retired after 45- years in the nuclear industry, plus ten years in teaching, I became a certified Yoga instructor in 2015. The engineering background let me appreciate India's ancient yogic wisdom traditions and their science. Yoga has survived for more than 5 000 years because it is logical and scientific.

In 2018, an opportunity came up to start the Sambandh yoga Gp for seniors in NJ. Members 55+ y/o have since been practicing with a purpose- to age gracefully and not be frail, not suffer from preventable chronic ailments, or not move into long-term care.

A retired grandpa, I am keeping excellent health, free of aches, Rx, or financial anxiety. My usual greeting style is - **Are You Yoging?** Not the outdated- How ye doin'?

Age is often highlighted in the Book to impress that anyone can be healthy without doing a challenging headstand, pretzel-like yoga pose, or taking more Rx. The secret is to live a yoga-based lifestyle, providing low or no-cost health insurance in the post-retirement golden years. Every asana, pranayama, or kriya in the Book is tested to be useful to seniors, not made-up

In America, the population of senior citizens is increasing at a faster rate than that of working-age adults. Therefore, healthy seniors are an issue of national importance because there is a distinct possibility of saving billions of dollars currently spent on their healthcare.

So, let's be friends with Yog and together impact the world in positive ways.

How did I Become a YOGA student?

- The fruit knows a tree it bears and the shade it provides to weary travellers. We choose what we sow, but we do not directly control how many fruits we will harvest. After landing in America in 1984, past the mid-age, my immediate goal was to remain healthy, take minimum time off from work, and establish the Rustagi family respectfully in a foreign land.

- My interest in yoga began with the 12 steps of Surya Namaskar, learned at a Hindu temple in NJ in 1985. However, the yearning was to enrol at an accredited yoga school in India.

Did curiosity turn me into a YOGA teacher?

- In 2013, I got a valuable sermon, 'Ravi, it is high time to learn how not to fall sick,' a short wise talk from my wife on her death bed. Nonetheless, I was also curious to improve my breathing, sharpen my mind, and hear the inner musical voice?

- I searched online for accredited yoga schools in India. Luckily, The Yoga Institute (TYI) in Santa Cruz East, Mumbai, accepted my enrolment in their 200-hour Teachers Training program in March 2015. The average age of 32 students in the class was 27 years, and I was 79.

- I continue to feel blessed that the short duration of yoga training in India was like my rebirth to study the super science of yoga, as significant as the science of nuclear fission. Both technologies lead from ignorance to knowledge, unreal to real. Interestingly, both sciences could be grafted as part of my daily life - one to earn a living, the other to live well.

The idea of writing the eBook- Yoga on Go?

- As a school student in India, it was my habit to make extensive notes from what the teacher spoke or wrote on the blackboard in the class. The habit of engaging the hands, the eyes, the minds, and assisting other students voluntarily has stayed with me ever since.

- The slides and stories presented in the Book are the triumph of an erstwhile shy, stuttering kid, now grown into a confident, healthy, senior citizen living in America.

PART ONE:

WHAT IS YOGA?

ACTS 1 - 12 ARE PRESENTED FOR SELF-STUDY

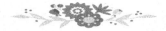

The human body has ten (10) openings: nine (9) to eliminate the stinky wastes, which is Nature's way to healthy living. (2 eyes, 2 ears, 2 nostrils, anus, regenerative organ, skin)

10 is the mouth - its purpose is to eat sensibly and speak softly.

TIP: Read body language on waking in the morning (happy or depressed) to choose the proper Asana.

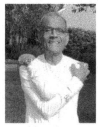

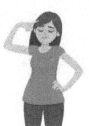

Happy   Depressed

Suryanamaskar in a chair prevents sickness and stagnation from catching up.

Hence, care for these new possibilities, & redeem rewards.

Reward 1: Every hour of physical exercise, like gardening, walking a dog, or jogging on the treadmill, can add up to 2 hours to your life.

Reward 2: Every hour of Yoga, uniting physical, mental, and spiritual bodies can add up to 5 hours.

Reward 3: A safety sign on NJ highway: 3-sec buckling up adds years to your life.

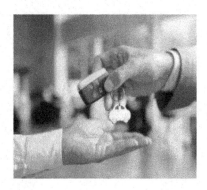

Treat Life as a holy contract from God, more than leasing a car from the car dealer. It is important to pay the lease rent on time and maintain the car as per the owner's manual. Else, the vehicle can be taken away, and the contract terminated prematurely.

IT'S COOL TO YOG: YOGA-ON-GO

Yoga takes us from unreal to Real, ignorance to Knowledge, death to Immortality

Practicing 3Rs as a habit will control not only the direct cause of *karma* in what you do, think, or speak but indirectly also the effect *karmaphala* (on-go progress)

-     R-1. Right intention (aim @ higher level)
-     R-2. Right breathing (deep/rhythmic)
-     R-3: Right posture (conscious of spine) [1]

[1] TIP: Most body pains are cured by correcting the physical posture R-2, plus Tadasana pose in twisting with chanting. You would feel instantly better. Add 20-min meditation to work fatigue-free during the day, and sleep well at night.

3Rs mean inseparability of the physical, mental and energy bodies in any act, Ex:

-     R-1 creates friendliness to self. Ex. gently smile, close the eyes, sit/stand relaxed in a favourite mudra, and chant in silence. Let this be your new ID.

- Even an indoor plant blossoms when relocated from the dark basement to the lighted yoga studio room near the window and in an upright orientation.

- A sissy dog behaves better when moved from a dog shelter to a regular home!

Face mask

- R-2 & R-3 help the body gain more strength, the mind thinks clearly, and healthy emotions rise in the heart, promoting fitness at all three levels.

Soon, you'll be seeing the bigger picture and moving from a short to a long-term goal. Ex.

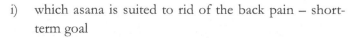

Indoor plant

i) which asana is suited to rid of the back pain – short-term goal

ii) acquire tools to calm the mind (chitta vritti nirodha [YS I.2])- long term goal [2]

[2] TIP: Ex. In Ramayana, Vibhishan chanted Ram's name in his home in Lanka and drew Hanuman's attention.

Ex. In the Kaun Banega Crorepati (KBC) TV show- often the player hurriedly makes a wrong decision and loses big money, treating precious life as a chance/gamble.

INTRO

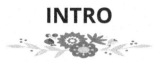

Yoga-On-Go is a practical tool to know that life's purpose is to rise from the basic survival mode: eat, sleep, reproduce, and die ~ 96 % of people to the higher thrive mode: mere live ~ 4 % of people meaningfully.

To progress from survive to thrive mode, the human mind performs four functions.

- - i) Manas (the basic memory) unconsciously stores impressions gathered by the five senses.
- - ii) buddhi (the physical intellect/conscious reasoning mind) is more concerned with facts and logical thinking. Impressions received from manas are now analysed for guidance/further action.

Un-conscious/
Semi-conscious mind

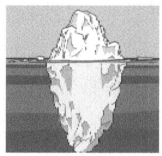

Sub-conscious
(hidden) mind

-iii) (a) Ahamkara (the -ve egoist vagrant mind) partners with lower intellect for more money and pleasures when life's goal is to do only what pleases the senses (survive mode). Most people function unaware of their higher potential, thrive mode (Ex: submerged part of an iceberg)

-iii) (b) svabhiman (the sub-conscious mind). A time comes in your sadhana when the limiting intellect ii) and ahamkara iii a) take a back seat. The creative subconscious Mind is prepared to sow quality seeds of peace, wisdom, and limitless prosperity.

-iv) Chitta (the deepest level of mind) This is the REAL mind, the ultimate Consciousness; it stays with you even after you die. Chitta is an unfettered, unprejudiced, ripple-free mind, partnering with cosmic and functions without an iota of memory. It also means access to the state of yoga, according to Indian sage Patanjali [YS1.2]

- Imagine yourself sitting under a tree, cool breeze blowing thru you, not around you. Now begin to control your thought processes through the powers invested in the subconscious mind. iii b

- Or, imagine you're an artist painting continuously. A calm Chitta surely produces quality work of art.

- My educational background in Newtonian and Quantum physics helps to appreciate the Maya, physically changing world of discrete objects vis-à-vis the invisible spiritual world of particle & wave energy.

TOTAL HEALTH, Inc.

Total Health begins with realizing that you are more than a physical being (you can see); you're also a mental being (you can feel, not see) and a spiritual being (not feel, nor see, only experience)

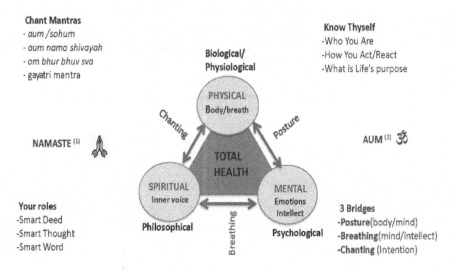

(1) NAMASTE is an ancient echo-friendly Hindu greeting, proclaiming we both are awesome, regardless of our age, religion, or status, that brings instant harmony among people.

(2) AUM is the shortest Vedic mantra, invoking Supreme power manifesting the entire universe. NAMASTE and AUM are the most straightforward sounds of yoga, it is no use shaking hands or kiss for a good morning.

SEVEN HABITS OF HEALTHY YOU

Health is beyond treating a disease; it is the prevention of disease

Body/Brain = sensing   Mind = thinking/deciding

Heart = innate intelligence   Soul = imperishable spirit)

Sl. No.	New habit	Ways/Means	Net gain
1	Body posture- be steady	Regular practice	Ache-free/fit body
2	Do not miss break-fast	Eat nutritiously	Good start to the day
3[1]	Breathe- slow/deep/rhythmic	Do pranayama	Begin inner journey
4	Mind quietens/emotions calm	Daily Yoga-on-go	A healthy body
5	Cultivate presence/ patience/ acceptance	Mindfulness-yoni mudra	Withdrawal of senses by *rechak kriya*
6	Discover the inner voice	*Abhyas/vairagya*[2]	Know what you're
7	*Chitta*- ripple-free *mind*	Continue meditation	Spiritual awakening

[1] Ex: If Breathing is shallow, the innate intelligence chooses the right *Pranayama.*

If posture is shaky, choose proper Asana, or the quality of stretching.

If you are in a bad mood, choose better breathing.

Soon, you're making better choices and exploring new territories

'Yoga On Go' attempts to nurture all seven habits of total health.

(2) *Abhya*s is to practice *dharma*, what upholds and *Vairagya* is to let-go *adharma what hurts.*

The mission: Technology and YOG are wonderful gifts to humanity.

Technology offers comfort, and YOG offers inner growth as well.

Together, you can fight terror, hunger, cancer, & COVID-19.

The world needs more than ever before: not too clever or intelligent people, but Yog-trained, intuitively smart students and teachers, retirees, and leaders.

YOGA IS A DISCOVERY

- The highest virtue of Yoga is

  i) physical movements are slow and harmonious,

  ii) mind and the body remain connected thru right breathing, and at the end, you feel not only energetic, but also joy blossoming in you.

- A yogi discovers that every cell in the body is engineered to be healthy. Furthermore, yoga creates the right environment appropriate for growth.

- This Book advocates a supreme healing approach that YOG is as indispensable as air, water, or food. With a higher population of yogis, there will be fewer crowds at the doctor's offices or in pharmacy stores and we will not have to build more hospitals.

- You'll not only live in the society but also realize two facts of meaningful living:

  1) you will not create obstacles for yourself, and

  2) you will not disturb others. Ex. Reclining the seat in the airplane so that the passenger behind you is not inconvenienced. You are then a cultured, mindful citizen, justifying the sacrifice in acquiring these better habits.

- London's Daily Telegraph 18-June-2019 reported 'Children of 6 years of age of divorced parents became obese and sick, because the single parents lived an unbalanced life, had less time to cook a healthy meal, and also had less money to buy fresh fruits or vegan'.

- Published Research shows that 1 in 3 adult males in America develop colorectal cancer if they have a family history. If discovered and treated in time, the 5-year survival rate is 90% or higher.

The end goal in yoga must be Samadhi (limb 8 of Ashtang yoga). To many, this is a challenging final step, like climbing Mt. Everest at 8,848 m altitude. Yet, it is okay to first reach the lower base, relax and get ready for the higher assault. Experienced mountaineers well versed in yoga first reach the EBC (Everest Base Camp) at 5,600 m and enjoy a stunning view before reaching the tallest peak in the world.

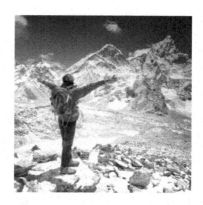

A great beginning!

- Formal weekly classes of the Sambandh Yoga Group began in 2018 in Livingston, NJ. Senior men and women have practiced for over 100 weeks-feeling more fit and more energetic.

- YOG or 'Yoga-On-Go' became a big draw- How to live healthy naturally, free of drugs/Rx?

Often, yoga is downgraded to 1-hour practice on specific days. YOG means no spiritual divide.

YOG encourages an 'out-of-box' approach, and you're not wasting energy on trivial issues. For example-

If you had an illness…	How did it heal itself, and you move on?
If your child was bullied in school…	How did you manage, causing no fight or insult?
If you had an issue with a neighbor…	How did you disagree and still held hands?
If an unhealthy dessert was served…	How did you satisfy the craving and not eat?

- YOG teaches: it is never too late, nor too early to re-train your faculties. Remember the slogan: use it or lose it.

Any meaningless rest (Krishna calls it akarma) and rust go together.

Ex: sing and cook work better as the brain-heart connection strengthens.

Sing & cook

TIP: The future holds promise to those Smarty ones who boldly affirm: I Yog

Aside! You can begin your casino experience entering the airport building by visiting Las Vegas.

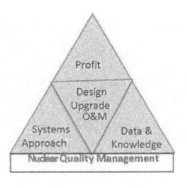

Airport Casino

Similarly, let your Yoga experience begin as you wake up in the morning or as soon as your limbs move, thoughts fly, or moods govern.

TOTAL QUALITY MANAGEMENT (TQM)

Total health is a multi-task effort

The integral concept of Health is making inroads in the industry, to reduce cost, upgrade design and improve profit and customer satisfaction.

Ex. TQM in nuclear power plants was started in the 1970s for Quality control during manufacture. Later, the idea spread to design engineering and

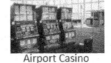

Profit

Design Upgrade O&M

Systems Approach

Data & Knowledge

Nuclear Quality Management

operation/maintenance over the 60-year operating life of the plant.

- Likewise, personal Health is more than doing routine exercise or brisk walking to burn calories to maintain body weight during holiday time.

- YOG is transforming- combining strength, empathy, & emotional intelligence.

  Ex. In charity donation, the heart decides if OK to give; let the mind decide how much?

  Then hands write the money check and legs walk to mail the envelope.

- YOG also confers good habits in a planned way and keeps the sickness/struggle at bay*

- Till the mid 20th century, the principal health slogan used to be:

  'Take care of mouth, eat bellyful, drink good wine, and you are in good health.'

- As understanding of the body-mind-soul/spirit connection progressed, the slogan has changed

  'Take Care of body/mind/breathing, and the trio is Total Health.'

*Hindi couplet- Dukh me simran sab kare, sukh me kare na koi. Jo sukhme me simran kare, to dukh kahe hoi.

- (Everyone prays when facing a hardship, but if you pray in good times, then hardship may not arise)

TIP: The hardships experienced in old age may be rooted in negligence in younger years.

A mechanical device needs a lubricant to overcome friction in moving parts.

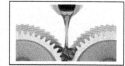

Lubricating oil
Or the soul spirit

In humans, the 'hidden' soul Spirit works as the silent lubricant when awakened.

- Every morning, say Namaste to anyone you meet, starting with yourself

- When upset, take a deep breath or two and avoid a hasty, wrong reaction.

- Every organ in the body likes to be healthy. By itself, an injured foot can't heal; it needs to summon a helping hand thru feeling in the heart. Here is the relevance of YOG and the power of simple asanas, manifesting like a lubricant to make life stress-free.

At the 2019 contest, the Jamaican beauty Ms. Toni Ann Singh won the Miss World title in London, U.K., on December 14, 2019, said, "Beauty was the least important personal aspect of my achievement."

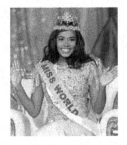

Ms. Tony A Singh

Ms. Singh, the first black woman to win the world title, added, "She wants to use her title to work for making sustainable change for women and children, and different values for life for the children and children's children."

She was looking ahead at the bigger picture and preparing to lead and guide the underprivileged children at her pace.

TIP: A costly exercise machine in a gym club may make you more efficient or burn more calories quicker. But YOG in your home setting ultimately makes you more relaxed, humane, and healthier. The asana in a yoga studio is to sync body, mind, and intellect to work as a coordinating team!

- Evolve means progressively rise from stage I (selfish) to stage II (unselfish) to stage III (selfless).

- **Ex.** If near a crime scene, a selfish simply watches and does nothing?

  A selfless citizen of the state, calls 911; it may save a life,

  and you're moving beyond, may grow into a superman.

- Blood is thicker than water- is a famous saying.

  It would mean building relations; the whole world is a family.

What can be nearer than physical body to mind, mind to breathing, and breathing connecting to intellect?

You get unexpected benefits as you sit, stand, walk, talk, eat, drink, study, work, drive, or relax, just by doing your acts in a yogic way.

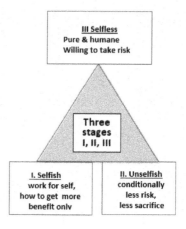

- As time passes, neighbours become friends, and friends become associates. You'll enjoy their social bonding and develop better habits. For example-

- Getting up for an appointment without an alarm clock, loving quiet moments, or hearing the inner voice

- Doing poses, asanas & kriyas, even during midnight hours.

- Unnoticed, you're evolving into a smart/human being, from selfish to selfless; that is transforming.

ACT-1: SIT STEADY & BE PAIN-FREE

Sitting in a convenient upright posture is the beginning of yoga

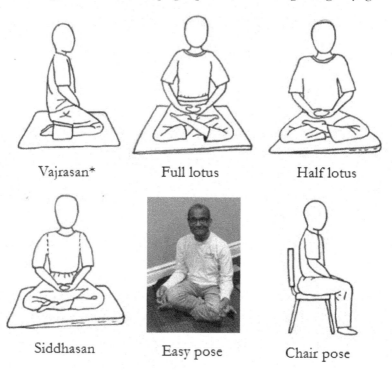

| Vajrasan* | Full lotus | Half lotus |

| Siddhasan | Easy pose | Chair pose |

Six (6) Good Meditative Postures

*TIP: Be creative-use a cushioned block or sit on one foot. Choose a meditative posture in which you remain awake, and with a tall spine.

- Sitting directly on the floor is preferred, as pressure on the pelvic bone is reduced because of the larger area under the legs, and you can meditate longer.
- Sitting upright in a cushioned chair, with each foot firmly on the floor, is a good alternative.

In each case, keep your fingers in a divine gesture, aka ***Mudra***

practice 3-in-1: act, breathe & chant in harmony

- upgrade your breathing rate ~ 10 breaths/min (sign of deep breathing)
- take a short break to control postural drift/fatigue

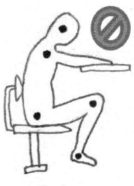

Bad pose

TIP: treat yourself as a ticketed passenger on a city bus; a steady posture is your ticket.

How many hours does an average American sit, stand, or walk besides sleeping?

Following is the result of a recent survey:

Sitting 13 hours; sleeping 8 hours; Total sedentary time 21 hours a day.

A new term 'Sitting disease' connotes a **sedentary** lifestyle, as this has a link with - diabetes, obesity, cancer, and cardiovascular diseases.

TIPS- To avoid neck/shoulder/back pain while working on your computer:

i)   Adjust the height of the computer screen such that the eyes can cover from top to bottom without having to strain the neck

ii) Take a break every 30 minutes to exercise your neck & shoulder for 30 seconds.

iii) Every hour, take a longer break for a 5-minute yogic walk.

•   If unable to walk, sit down in a meditative pose and imagine you're doing an Asana.

Inhale to be in the posture. Exhale to picture yourself returning to the starting position.

This is the power of visualization, aka the resolve/intent #1 of 3Rs.

Also, try to engage the 5 cognitive senses, and notice the internal and external sights and sounds-

level, nature, and pitch, how these come and go, and observe your own witnessing in effect?

• Six sitting postures are technically called: *Asanas for pranayama and meditation*:

Padmasan (full lotus), **Ardh padmasan** (half-lotus), **Siddhasan** (the accomplished posture)

Vajrasan (the hero posture) is good for digesting food, & **Sukhasan** (easy pose)

Chair posture is for those who feel better than sitting on the floor for an extended time.

TIP: Your favourite pose is one in which you can sit steady for 20 or more minutes [YD 2.46]

ACT- 2: PREVENT FALLS

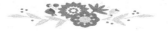

Two Leading Causes of Falls in senior citizens

Cause 1. Incorrect Posture

Remedy: Work or stand in a balanced posture, with neck and spine aligned

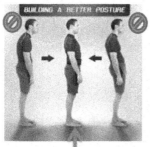

Good posture

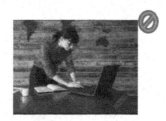

.... Bad work posture...........
shoulder, & upper back
are stressed

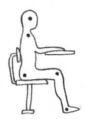

Good posture

Typing hurriedly, standing, and sipping coffee at the same time are bad habits, a grave risk is causing pain to the lower/upper back.

Typical pain areas are: Shoulder 38%, Neck 53%, Waist 33%, Low back 63%

Net Result: Follow 3Rs; you have the skill to convert a dull chore into a healthy yogic act.

- The good news: 96% of Americans would be willing to stand or walk longer to improve their health and life expectancy.

- Falls are a hidden epidemic among people of all ages; 6 out of 10 falls occur in homes.

- Dangerous falls are preventable with the following simple measures

i) When changing the posture- from sitting to standing/walking – take time to scan the ground ahead for a pitfall

ii) There is a healthy way to stand, resulting in the minimum bulge at the waist

iii)   Both feet share 50 – 50% load, and toes point forward.

iv)   Also, wear the right shoes, & remove tripping/falling/slipping hazards, such as rugs, furniture, clutter, water spill in walkways

v)   must use night lights in bedrooms, bathrooms, and hallways, or carry with you in your suitcase when sleeping over with friends/relatives

vi)   In the shower area, keep a chair to sit on and use a non-slip mat.

vii)   Pranayama in hot/humid air in the bathroom is the antidote to mucus formation.

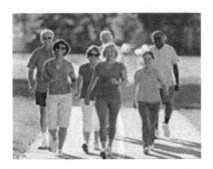

Walking Club

viii)   Join a Walking Club to enjoy the fun of being outdoors

ix)   Have your vision, hearing, and diagnostics checked regularly.

Finally, talk to your doctor about the side effects of the Rx medication if you're taking.

Next is Cause 2 of Falls

Cause 2. Ineffective Use of Brain

Remedy: Coordination- Let eyes follow the feet as you move

Safe standing:

keep feet parallel, a foot apart, arms folded, in front or on back; both postures keep you slouch-free, avoiding drooping shoulders

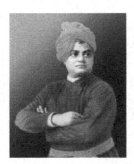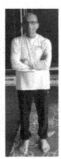

Stand safe in style

Safe walking:

First, scan the ground ahead for a pothole or obstruction, then get up to walk forward

**Body/mind disconnected
Unsafe walking**

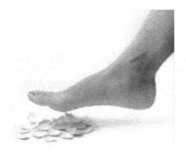

Safe picking up:

Scan the height for safe reach, then use a step stool/support

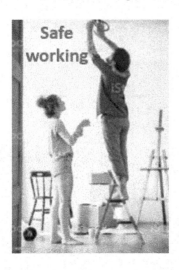

Stay relaxed, use the 30-30 rule*,

*Every 30 min, take a 30-sec break- tense and relax the body, and look away from the computer screen cures eye/neck fatigue

Standing tall is symbolic of strength, stability, and willpower.

• Doesn't a baby feel great as she learns how to stand up on her own?

• Modern Americans, 90% of them are willing to stand longer and work, as it improves their life expectancy, at no extra cost.

• Children don't need reasoning, as they breathe deep naturally

• An adult needs proof, written evidence because he is disconnected from his inside Reality.

• It is easy to stand tall in the Tadasana pose when the spine is kept upright.

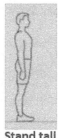

Stand tall

Besides, try variants of this easy posture to do more challenging roles

- Burn extra calories

- Tone muscles

- Improve balance

- Increase blood flow to painful spots

- Reduce blood sugar levels, and

- Ramp up metabolism

When you begin to ask open questions -

Who is God?   Who am I?   Where do I go from here?

You rise above the dogmas and rituals; your approach is meaningful beyond making a comfortable living.

There are less than 5% of people whose goal is to live meaningfully.

Being conscious of the minutes and seconds, you learn the discipline of not wasting anything worthwhile - material goods, food, breaths, and the limited time on earth.

- Begin with your worst habit, hurting you most of the time, ex—poor posture, judging/maligning others. **Soon, you're catching up on more habits, including getting rid of a lingering negative mindset.**

- **Were these waiting for your yogic lifestyle?** *Answer: emphatically is YES.*

Simple Exercise for Better Posture....

- Stand with knees slightly bent to avoid locking

- Heels firm on the ground and 15-cm away from the wall

- Slide up/down in slow motion, keeping the head, shoulders, and butts in contact with the wall

- Feel stretch in thigh muscles, which are meant to provide for strong knees, as the knees do not have a muscle. **If you have knee pain,** the muscles in the shin or thigh need strengthening. I tried more, but this is the best.

- Repeat 20X in 2 minutes to build optimum quad strength.

- **TIP**: If a vertical wall is not handy, you may sit or stand upright while stretching both arms upward during inhaling.

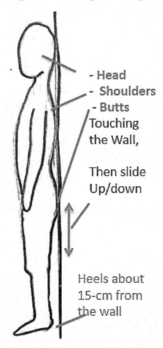

- Head
- Shoulders
- Butts
Touching
the Wall,

Then slide
Up/down

Heels about
15-cm from
the wall

Try with one hand at a time, then switch to both arms.

TIP: Simple exercises 30 sec each- improve posture on the go, from computer work.

1. Stand similar to Talasan. Raise your hands and stretch in inhale.

2. Clasp your hands on your back, and stretch as far back comfortably.

3. Lie down on the floor, keep the cushioned pillow under your back

More Tips On – Standing Posture

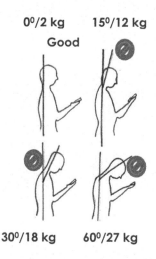

0°/2 kg   15°/12 kg

Good

30°/18 kg   60°/27 kg

Easy Exercises To Help Prevent Falls

Use a chair if needed

- **Weight Shifting** – Standing, shift weight to one side and hold foot off floor for up to 30 seconds.

- **One-Legged Balancing** – Standing, lift one foot, bending at knee. Hold up to 30 seconds.

- **Heel-Toe Walk** – Take 10-20 steps, placing the heal of one foot directly in front of other foot.

- **Leg Raises** – While sitting, extend one leg in front of you and hold for one second. Repeat 10-15 times, then switch legs.

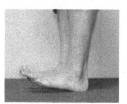

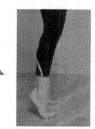

ACT- 3: WALK FATIGUE-FREE

Acknowledge the whole you: hands, feet, eyes, breath, chant, & smile

you can walk longer/faster & fatigue-free

Suggested 30-min. yogic walk combo covers 1-mile, burns 100 -Cal, or more

8-min slow walk +	8-min medium walk +	14-min brisk walk =	30-min total walk
4 steps/6-sec	4 steps/3-sec	4 steps/2-sec	1.1 mi
1 mph	2 mph	3 mph	110 Cal

GOOD STYLE: torso upright,
Heel or sole contact ground

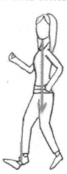

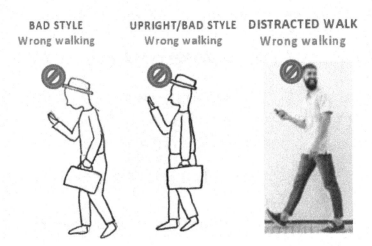

BAD STYLE	UPRIGHT/BAD STYLE	DISTRACTED WALK
Wrong walking	Wrong walking	Wrong walking

Scan the ground ahead before getting up from your seat

Always keep inhale = exhale, and **do not attempt advanced Pranayama kriya in walking**

Bonus: conscious walk auto-corrects body posture, improves bone strength & balance

CHAIR-WALKING & MARCH-IN-PLACE

Relaxing alternatives, while watching TV, or taking a break

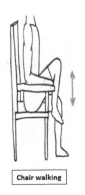

BOTH FEET FIRM ON GROUND, PARALLEL AND A FOOT APART

KEEP YOUR BACK ERECT, UNSUPPORTED & SHOULDERS RELAXED

CHANT *SOHAM* **MANTRA**
INHALE & EXHALE
MOVE/CYCLE LEGS UP & DOWN
DO 10-20 SETS IN 2 - 4 MINUTES
rhythmically breathing & moving

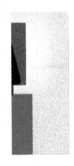

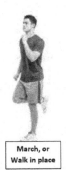

March, or
Walk in place

Chair walking

Note-1: You can practice more Asanas on a chair, for Ex: Surya namaskar

Note-2: March in place, a speed increase of 10% heals the heart, improves mood, and reduces pain in the neck/back, hence strongly recommended for seniors. More so, it preferentially loads the sole.

Note-3: For multiple benefits- coordinate blinking of eyes, breathing, chanting, and smile

Note-4: The chair must be hard, without arms, and with a soft cushion.

MAKE REVERSE WALKING a New Hobby

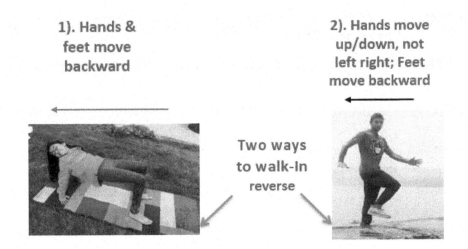

1). Hands & feet move backward

2). Hands move up/down, not left right; Feet move backward

Two ways to walk-In reverse

Walking in reverse is beneficial to physical and mental well-being.

Challenges different muscles in hands & legs,

Cultivates balance, knee health, cardio-fitness, and mental function. 'Let Go' boredom in life, as muscles enjoy the freedom to do 'Tapas' their way.

Don't we do *Viprit Karni, Sarvangasana* poses in reverse?

Try Reverse Counting 10 – 1 or 20 - 1 in one inhale, or one exhale to improve mental focus.

Ex. Jeopardy game, Reverse Engineering, Reverse Mortgage

Enjoy paying attention to the inside as a Spiritual hobby of reversing

WALKING/STANDING WITH HANDS BEHIND

- Walking in reverse, as shown, is an option to be safe and fun at your own pace.

- This is wonderful learning, as you can coordinate your move, chanting, and rhythm in reverse. Also, it keeps the brain healthy.

- Observe how walking in reverse feels different than walking forward. You will marvel because you can't just walk- in reverse without being fully aware of your body and the environment.

- Alternatively, take a break, try walking, or marching consciously with hands behind, holding a fist in other hands.

  After eating, walk-in this mode for 10 minutes instead of sitting down to work.

  You will instantly feel better and ready to get back to work.

- Your true North remains focused on the job at hand.

- You would like to walk 'consciously' more often, making it your default mode.

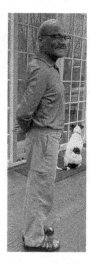

TIP-1: Make your feet feel good when your mind doesn't feel good. Give a complimentary massage to the feet. Soon, the mind gets the relief signal.

TIP-2: The body/mind is a storehouse of free Apps; download these.

\-   Try walking on a Tread Mill in the comfort of your home or a sports club. Treat the Treadmill as a Yogic accessory.

\-   I love it because the final numbers are displayed: 3 mph, 3% incline, 150 calories, in 2 km, in 30 minutes.   – Use the 3Rs throughout to suit your capacity.

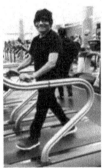

Tread mill

\-   If you live near the sea, run barefoot on the beach, and start the loving feel of mother earth caressing your feet. Like a baby anxiously learning to walk, you will want to do an intelligent yogic walk more often for 20 min non-stop. Within a few weeks, you will experience a surge of energy in your heart and strength in your legs.

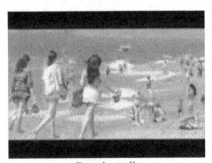

Beach walk

The phrase 'Survival of the Fittest' is strictly the law of the jungle for the survival of animals but is wrongly applied to preserving favoured races among humans.

In Yog, fitness means every person has been gifted with raw skills and divine energy. When you learn how to utilize that energy, anyone prospers, even if handicapped.

WALKING MEDITATION

It is a cruel fact that gravity takes over as you age. Unless you get fun slowing down, shaking legs, swinging hands, combining walking and chanting, exploring a new you, you are liable to fall.

i) Bend arms 90o,   ii) swivel hips,

iii) shoulders, knees, ankles aligned   iv) heel/toe in rhythm

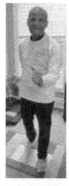
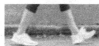

Benefits: Know thy self	Feel good instantly	Increase lifespan
Prevent heart disease	Control high B.P.	Manage diabetes
Improve memory, sleep better	Better breathing	Right posture
Relieves body pain, and fatigue	Trim the waist	Enhanced energy

You can customize walking meditation….

Gayatri's mantra is 2 lines, 16 words, and 4 parts. To derive its benefit in walking, walk briskly and chant 150X in 20-minutes. Inhale/exhale rhythmically, chant 4 words/4 steps in each breath.

1. Aum.Bhur.Bhuva.Svah-	Oh God! the giver of life, remover of pains, & bestower of happiness.
2. Tat.Savitur.Vare.Nyam-	Thou are luminous, pure, and adorable
3. Bhargo.Devasya.Dhi.Mahi-	We meditate on thee. May thou guide
4. Dhiyo.YoNah.Pracho.Dayat-	our intellect in the right direction

Note 1: Significance of Gayatri mantra – God shows the way, but picking up speed is human effort.

Note 2: You chant - Aum1, Aum2, Aum3, Aum4 consciously- rather than 1, 2, 3, 4 mechanically

Note3: Brisk pace - 3 mph speed, 1 mi distance, 150 chants in 20 min, 100 calories

Medium pace - 2 mph speed, 0.6 mi distance, 100 chants in 20 min, 50 calories

Slow pace - 1 mph speed, 1/3 mi distance, 50 chants in 20 min, 25 calories

ACT- 4: BEND & LIFT SAFE

4-stages:

i) sit, slouch-free

ii) begin stand, look ahead

iii) stand up,

iv) keep head, back, butts aligned

Anti-aging line/flat back

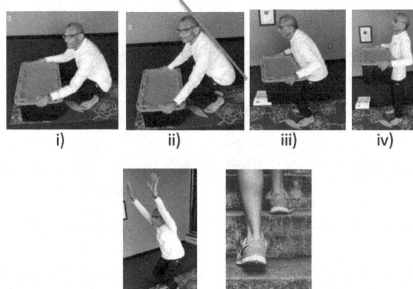

i)   ii)   iii)   iv)

Utkatasan

Climb Stair
Bend the good leg

TIP: For safe bending/lifting/twisting, consider the body as a lever

-     Decide the fulcrum pivot which does not move, say the hip joint

-     Then, the two arms of the lever and the body move as a unit

-     The anti-aging line maintains for flatback

-     Observe better breathing when twisting

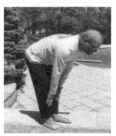

Bend at hip, upper torso behaves as one unit

TWIST SAFE

Twist and exhale go together. Split a long exhale inconvenient step.

Let the exhaling start from the abdomen and end in the chest area.

Inhale on return in one step of 2-3 sec

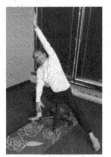 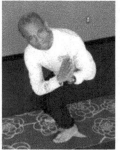

Trikonasan (Triangle pose)   Twisted side angle pose

> ***TIP:*** *YOG helps to improve your attitude-Yogic twisting/ bending works wonders. Like growing a kitchen garden, you will be thrilled to notice a chain of benefits- better BP, bodyweight, etc. Overall, humbler and more adaptable.*

Key movements in the twisted pose are- axial body & spinal extension. Twisting safely has the potential to keep the lower back in good shape, with a lesser risk of spine hardening and fusing in senior years. **Twisting & exhaling provide instant energy, as better breathing is restored.**

TIP: If twisting the upper torso is not easy, first move one foot.

ACT- 5: BREATHE BETTER

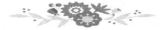

A businessman cares for every penny,

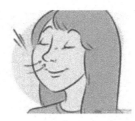

Yogi cares for every breath: honor thy breath, enjoy thy life

Breathing 101- Let us refresh the basics

- Your first Inhale at birth and the final exhale at death- both are not in your control

- Yet millions of breaths in between are in your control; yoga teaches how you may feel accomplished making a trip to holy Kailash?

Mount Kailash

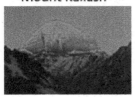

Breathing Statistics

- Good healthy breathing 15 breaths/min (bpm), or 21,600 breaths in a day

- Better breathing 12 bpm, or 17,000 breaths in a day

- Yogic breathing < 10 bpm. (inhale + exhale = 6 sec) *

- Air inhaled @15 bpm ~ 10,300 liters of air in a day to feed trillions of cells in the chest

- Chest expansion %: exhale to inhale (4% healthy/< 2% sign of sickness)

What more can better Breathing do for you?

- Breathing is your most precious gift. You can take it to a higher level, i.e., slow and rhythmic increases your healthy life span. It is a skill everyone can acquire through daily yoga.

- Make better breathing your permanent Armor, like the bow/arrow was to Sri Ramchandra during the 14-year exile.

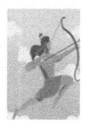

Rama, Bow/arrow

Seniors can improve their lung capacity with asanas that need twisting ex. Trikonasan.

*Cross 10 bpm barrier for wellness. This needs training and patience.

Try to focus on the subtle silence between inhale/exhale, and watch the joy erupting.

TIP: Gradually, you discover the bigger role of better breathing than a better body

THE GOOD Vs. BAD BREATHING

Breathing is an act you can change voluntarily; better breathing heals, cleanses, and nourishes

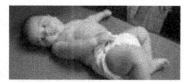

Baby breathes deep in belly

I.   Abdominal(deep/diaphragmatic), belly Breathing is slow and better

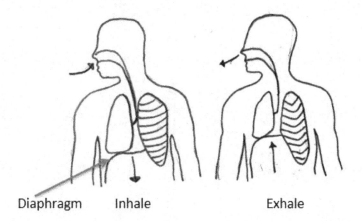

Diaphragm   Inhale   Exhale

- Inhales more oxygen to lungs and   more toxins out in exhaling

- steadies and calms the Mind

- the simplest way to live consciously

II.   Shallow (chest) bad breathing is fast and erratic

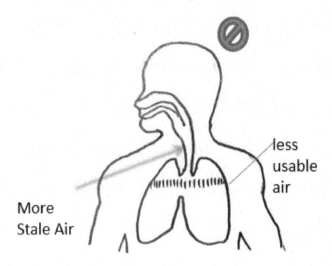

More
Stale Air

less
usable
air

- Sufficient oxygen is not fed to the body also enough toxins are not removed

- Trigger stress/anxiety/fatigue syndrome

- unaware of the nasal congestion

FIVE SIMPLE AND EFFECTIVE BREATHING EXERCISES

The following exercises are recommended for improved breathing (**practice in sitting/lying**)

- **Exercise 1:** *Jal Neti* cures nasal irrigation and personal hygiene to remove any debris or mucus from the nasal cavity, and breath can flow properly. Take a *neti* pot filled with warm saltwater. Pour the saline solution in one nostril at a time. The solution will flow out through the other nostril. Doing this *kriya* each morning and night frees you from colds, headaches, and infections.

- **Exercise 2:** Test your lung capacity- Inhale, hold, & Exhale- a total 30 sec or more is healthy lungs

- **Exercise 3:** Advanced deep breathing. Sit steady, eyes closed, on a chair or floor. Exhale through both nostrils, and be as relaxed/motionless as possible. Apply root lock by contracting rectum muscles. Continue exhaling, no exertion. Having exhaled completely, start inhaling slowly through the nostrils; try inhaling a little more after reaching the top. Repeat 10 cycles daily for 1-2 months. It is beneficial for curing BP and insomnia. This is more advanced deep breathing than P4

- **Exercise 4:** Another easier option is to lie on your back, palms on the upper abdomen, between the rib cage and the navel. Inhale/exhale through the nostrils slowly, smoothly, and fully. There should be no noise, jerks, or pauses in breathing to observe diaphragm function in 5-6 sec.

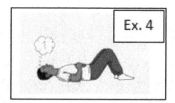

- **Exercise 5:** *Viprit karni* (legs up the wall pose) would help de-congest the mouth and nose and restore blood circulation through the head and heart. May use a cushion below the lower back for spine health and better lymph flow.

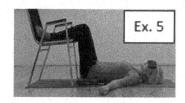

TIP: Better breathing should be introduced into the school curriculum.

Three more Rules of Better (slower) Breathing: how to inhale, exhale, and retain?

- **RULE 1: INHALE** while the body extends, such as rising or bending backward (lungs need more space), mentally affirm a mantra, and gaze at the eyebrows.

- **RULE 2: EXHALE** while the body contracts, such as bending forward, twisting, or sitting down (emptying the lungs is easier), and do

Root lock. Smile N Exhale...... A simple logic: **SMILE and STRESS do not co-exist**

- **RULE 3:** Break a complex asana pose into smaller steps. Ex. If a twist takes > 4 sec, split in 2 moves (2 breaths, each of 2 sec).

- The above 3 breathing Rules, plus meditation practice (ACT-12), are known as the gateway to consciousness.

- The Exhale/ Inhale combo is linked in the **Dog-Cat**, the **Wind Release pose**, or the **smile pose**. Practice these safe asanas often.

Dog/Cat pose

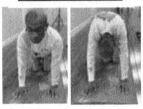

Gas release pose

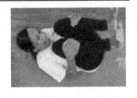

Smile pose

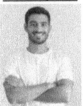

- **Caution:** Do not overstimulate the body thru fast or excessive breathing, except in advanced Pranayamas P-5 thru P-10, in the care of a yoga therapist.

- **TIP:** Right posture plus right breathing (slow and deep) through the nostrils is the foundation of yoga. You'll be amazed that a healthy breathing rate of 5-6 BPM can be accomplished in yogic breathing.

This conserves the allotted number of breaths and increases lifespan. Simultaneously, you are healing the age-related prostate as well as ego issues.

Better breathing con't

1. Pranayama is a Sanskrit term of two words: **Prana + Ayama**. **Prana** means the life force. **Ayama** means to control, mainly slowing down. Pranayama is the science of better breathing- deep, slow and mindful.

    At the basic level, breathing keeps you alive by bringing in oxygen, inhaling, and throwing out toxins exhaling. Advanced pranayamas nourish the body in a controlled manner, opening the pathway to higher Consciousness.

2. Healthy better breathing is a 3-part process

    - filling/inhaling (*purak*), continuous, jerk-free, and through the nose

    - emptying/exhaling (*rechak*), to be the same quality and duration as inhaling   holding breath kumbhak kriya are of two kinds- the inside (*antarik kumbhak* **holding breath in**) and the outside (*bahya kumbhak* **holding breath out**).

3. While extended *kumbhak* is not recommended in the initial stages, notice the brief natural silence after inhaling and exhaling. In that silence, stay quiet for a second. Repeat 10X. This practice will bring in deep relaxation, a natural antidote to hypertension.

4. Make better breathing your new lifestyle- your road to longevity. Ex: in marketing: Customer assistance is a phone call away. **A yogi says:** that *peace of mind is a deep breath away.*

5. In conclusion, pranayama and better breathing create a strong foundation for your health.

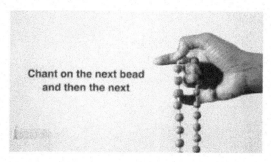

This aspect is covered in the next topic, **ACT-6** Techniques of Pranayama.

ACT- 6: TECHNIQUES OF PRANAYAMA

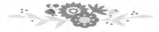

Don't Leave Home without the basic P1, P2, P3, and P4

P1	P2

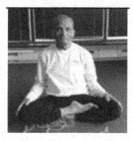 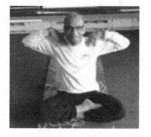

Voluntary Breathing
Live by choice

Clavicular Breathing
Clear the throat

- Sit steady, Check both nostrils are flowing equal. 3X

- Make right choices- fingers in gyan mudra, arms on thighs, eyes closed

- Inhale/exhale 3-sec each.

- Repeat 10 cycles.

Do Nadi Shodhan pranayama P5 modified, If nostrils are blocked.

- Keep fingers on collar bone, Inhale in 3 sec raising elbows, & collar bones together

- Exhale in 3 sec, lowering elbows & collar bones.

- Observe flow gushing thru throat, mucus flows out

- Repeat 10 cycles

P3

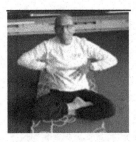

Shallow breathing
Expand the lungs

P4

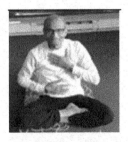

Deep breathing
Bring calmness

- Keep the two fore fingers between the ribs, left and right hands as shown.

- Inhale slow in 3-sec, or more till the fingers slide out fully

- Exhale in same time as inhale, fingers slide back in

- Observe the chest expanding, yet abdomen is steady

- Repeat 10 Cycles

- Inhale thru nose slow & deep, diaphragm moves down, belly expands. Allow breath to settle in the lower belly.

- Exhale slow, diaphragm moves up, belly contracts

- Inhale/exhale in steps is deep breathing.

- Repeat 10 cycles

ADVANCED PRANAYAMA P5, P6, P7, P8, P9, P10

Common to each Pranayama is the mental recitation of AUM, then the physical consciousness elevates to serve the higher Consciousness

P5- Nadi Shodhan

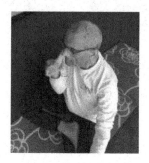

Purifies 72000 nerves

One nostril inhales/the other exhales

Start inhaling thru the left nostril

- Followed by exhaling thru right. Continue left/right process 3X

- After 3X, change the sequence

- Exhale thru right nostril,

- and inhale thru left. Do 3X

- This is one cycle- Repeat 2 more cycles at a stretch

Nadi shodhan:

With practice, add root lock, & retain the inhaled breath for 2-sec. Repeat 30X.

P6- Anulom Vilom

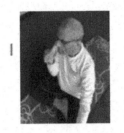 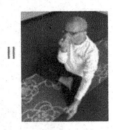

Alternate nostril breathing

The same nostril inhales, & exhale

Balances both hemispheres of the brain

- Begin exhaling slowly thru the left nostril in 3-sec, keeping the right nostril closed (I)

- Close the left nostril, open the right nostril, and inhale in 3-sec (II).

- Exhale thru right nostril in 3-sec

- followed by inhaling thru the left nostril

- Repeat 7- 21 full cycles and end in inhaling thru the left nostril.

Note: With practice, increase the speed, & repeat 100 cycles, directing the inhaled current to the Root chakra.

P7- Bhramari (Bee breath)

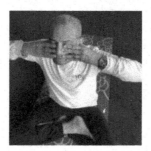

Improves voice & immunity

Applies brakes to the buzzing mind

- Inhale, gently close ears with thumbs, index fingers on eyebrows, middle fingers on the nose bridge, ring and little fingers on lips, eyes turned up & focused on Ajna chakra

- With your nose partially open, exhale slowly in a soft humming bee sound. Repeat min 21X till ready for yoni-mudra

Yoni mudra *Increases your willpower*

- narrow nasal passages by middle fingers.

- Equalize Inhale/Exhale for 5-8 sec, without the bee sound.

You may hear the inner voice of yourself

P8 - BRAHM KRIYA

Bhastrika variant

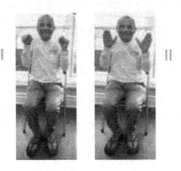

Boosts immunity

Courtesy, Manav Mandir Mission, Delhi

- Make a fist in both hands. I

- Start inhaling and opening fists in 1.5 sec. II

- Exhale fast in ½ sec, and re-close fists. Hold for 3 sec.

- This is 1 cycle. Do 10 cycles

- Take 2-3 deep breaths (P4).

  This is one set. Do 2 more sets.

- Repeat 2X in a day.

P9 – KAPALBHATI

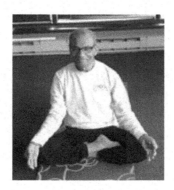

Breath of fire

Forehead shines

- Exhale deep vigorous thru nose, followed by relaxing abdominal muscles effortless or, Inhaling spontaneously.

- This is 1 cycle. Repeat 21X in quick succession

- In 1 month, an increase to 51 cycles

- has therapeutic value for diabetes, obesity, immunity, and constipation

P10 - PURSED LIPS

1:2 Breathing

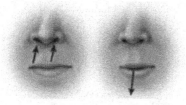

Inhale thru nose 2 counts

Exhale thru the mouth 4 counts

Benefits: Inhale thru the nose, and exhale thru the mouth with pursed lips, controls BP, relieve pulmonary issues, & promotes weight loss;

-do 5-10X without holding.

Caution: Be patient in building up inhale/exhale breathing ratio; It may hurt if forced.

Caution: consult the doctor, if you have a medical issue in the lungs, ear, and eyes

ACT- 7: BE CALM, & FOCUSED

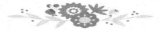

More than 80% of chronic diseases are artificial due to wrong beliefs

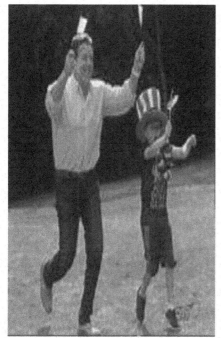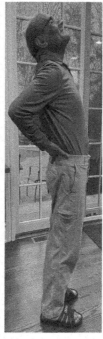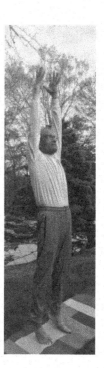

Dance & Share Your Smiles   *Tadasan variant*   *Talasan*

- **Tadasan pose:** Stand, feet together, keep eyes open, toes open, Inhale to focus on raising hands in 3-sec, and be careful not to fall. Hold 6 sec.

- Keep equal 50-50 pressure on each leg, giving you a sense of rootedness. In the **Talasan pose**, reaching the ceiling above will further tense the body. Exhale to return hands/toes close while stress dumps into the ground.

- Inhaling & exhaling with a smile in 3-sec each, and repeat 4- 5 times.

- **Option**: You may as well dance in the town park and smile the worries away

Instinct vs. reasoned intelligence?

Humans can use their experience and organized intelligence to modify their responses to certain stimuli. Ex. on the 9-11-2001 terror attack in New York, the people who escaped death were those lucky ones who acted instinctively and ran down the stairs or elevator without waiting to hear detailed instructions. Only 16-1/2 minutes were available to get out to safety!

For Instant relief: Tadasan variant heals the body pain, and Talasan pose dumps mental stress to the ground

The human body is widely acknowledged as the most sophisticated device, with trillions of cells, thousands of nadis, hundreds of bones, and visible or invisible body parts functioning without resting.

Another shocker! According to NASA researchers, you've 7 million times more atoms in your body than there are stars in the universe.

- For upkeep of the body, it is important to receive expert recharging and refreshing online- by proven yogic kriyas

  [Take the example of the KAIGA nuclear power plant in the Karnataka state of India. In this advanced indigenous design, nuclear fuel is loaded and used fuel removed daily while the plant is operating at 100% power. The KAIGA unit-1 established a World Record for the longest continuous run of 941 days in 2019]

KAIGA NPP, INDIA

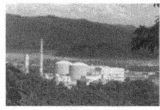

- The Tadasan pose , the three points in the foot remain firm on the floor; in Talasan , feet rise; both help removes the body fatigue on demand.

- Observe the strength gained as you put your whole weight on the left foot, then shift to the right foot, and vice-versa.

- Your effectiveness adds up each time you do the Tadasan/Talasan combo set. **Start to inhale (3 sec), hold (6 sec), exhale/smile (3 sec). In yog mudra pose, these numbers increase to make you feel good.**

- Similar happy feelings are experienced every morning, as the bowels move smoothly, followed by the Purity practice (pg. 87) in the shower room.

TIP: Simple recipe to ease nervousness (boredom-free living) is a 10-min sequence

i)   sit, stand, and observe 3Rs

ii) do basic four pranayamas P1 to P4

iii) do Tadasan plus Talasan poses in 3-6-3 sec

iv) give acupressure treatment on the back of the toes

v)   celebrate healing, and sharing with other body parts- you'll have more opportunities to feel good

TAKE A SABBATICAL

You can make the 3rd Niyama of 'Tapas'* more creative

On a festival time, such as the Ekadashi- the 11th lunar day of the month

TIP: Join with family/friends because Yoga means to unite for self and collective care.

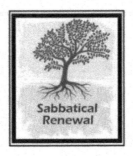

- Eat sattvik (delicious, fresh, gently spiced, vegan food), & avoid CRAP

  C=carbonated soda, R=refined oil or grains, A=added sugar, P=processed/stale food

- Take a hot bath, give massage to the body, and Do Yogasanas (choices

- Read a best seller, listen to music, paint, sing to the heart, Meditate, and get a glimpse of your higher reality?

- Surround yourself in a smart lifestyle- be a smart (Samarth) seeker, sleep in a smart, clean bed, breathe pollution-free air, and maintain social distancing

- Simultaneously, practice what helps (abhyas) & 'let go' what hurts (vairagya).

- Such meaningful habits can change the ABCD image of an Indian-American

from *America Born Confused Deshi* to *America Born Chatur Deshi*

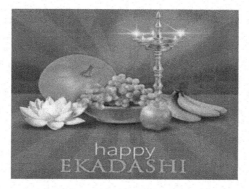

*(moral observances/austerities purify the body/mind/soul)

The sabbatical facility in higher colleges and universities lets the senior, tenured professors take a break from routine teaching and spend weeks and months on new research and higher learning.

A similar time off from the daily grind, even once a year, lets the householder aspire for higher goals and invite neighbors and friends from the local community?

BG Ch. 18 clarifies there are three cleansing acts (Yajna, Daan, Tap-oblations, charities, and austerities), which must not be relinquished even by a sanyasi (dissociated from worldly affairs) because these three satvik acts are a means of purifying you inside out.

Practice Tapas: in Sanskrit, Tapas means Heat, a trial application of purifying fire. Once you have successfully passed this test, you will overcome other barriers in the journey.

It is also necessary that the usual business-- money-making, gossiping, or pursuing material objectives- stops, as Ekadashi is observed for self-study and introspection.

Just for one Ekadashi 11th day in the lunar month, re-think Tapas, attaining higher freedom.

No 'junk' food + no 'junk' anxiety. Consider ending the day with the Yagna havan ritual for a better experience.

Such smart fasting goes above and beyond; it cleanses the stomach and purifies the mind.

TIP: To be a smart grandparent, try the following guidelines-

I.   When to take retirement? Plan for retirement when still healthy and financially ready to move into *vanaprastha* (a stage of progressive detachment).

II.   Pre-requisite to retire? Join a boot camp- a month or more- in a serene *ashram* setting; learn what self-healing is, with little or no dependence on Rx.

III. Where to retire? If you can afford it, live independently in a home suiting your current needs. You will make new friends too.

IV.   How to spend time? Plan to spend one or more months annually with the grandkids, to pass on the family traditions. Your priority always must be growth and learning, besides keeping good health.

Conclusion: GOOD (habits) + OLD (age) = GOLD....makes retirement years truly golden.

You'll live life meaningfully and be ready to die fearlessly. (Per Mahamrutnjya mantra)

ACT- 8: THE POWER OF POSITIVE

Yoga teaches +ve, how or what can you do better?

Yoga Sutra II.33 Vitark Baadhne Pratipaksh Bhavnam means 'When perverse thoughts inhibit yogic progress, the opposite should be considered. i.e., Lovingly

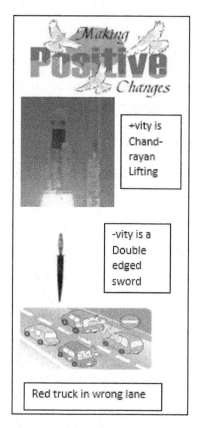

BG 17.3 yo yac-chraddah sa eva sah, let your faith be full of devotion, then mind thinks positive, and intellect prompts you to perform your favorite pose, dispelling the root of negative thinking.

Consider two +ve acts together for a stronger faith and better outcome. Ex. If gloomy rain is forecast, carry an umbrella & pray for better weather. Then your +ve aura expands, and your inner booster rocket Chandrayan lifts! A simple logic: Positive action produces a positive reaction.

- Treat negativity as erroneously driving in the wrong lane or as a 2-edge sword- hurting you twice as you act and again as he reacts in revenge. Hence, In retired living, try to kill two birds with one stone- by *abhyas* and *vairagya*.

Pay attention that struggles and lessons go together. A +ve person cares for the lesson and learns wisdom; a -ve person cares for hurt and suffers more.

- Ex. When in pain, say: 'There are a few things I can still do, despite my pain.' Instead of saying, 'I can't do it because the pain is killing me.'

Pessimism/worrying, on the contrary, robs your inbuilt defence mechanism, and you are unable to help yourself or any other'. In the ancient Vedas of India, there is a health Law- Worrying speeds up aging. Learn from your body- **A hand is ready to heal the foot or scratch the inaccessible upper back without worrying about return favor.**

- Optimism is the urge of all seekers. Optimistic people are known to accomplish more and suffer less. 'A glass-half-full with water and another half with air' is better than saying only 50% full, 50% empty, so says India's PM Narendra Modi.   Out-of-box thinking conveys the idea of making you aman, no-mind or thoughtless, overcoming meaningless fault finding/worldly desires.

> I. Routine thinking:
> - Half full/half empty
> II. Out-of-box thinking:
> - Half air/half water

- I met a centenarian, George Klein (b. Feb 11, 1920), resident of Livingston, NJ, going strong at 100+; he attributes his long life to optimism and volunteering. 'Optimism attracts more people, and no one likes to associate with the negative-minded, crying, complaining, and comparing folks' he said: Some memory loss with age is inevitable, yet a positive mindset stops the rapid loss.

- Similarly, it is your smart duty to do dishes, as dishes have a right to look their best. Then, it will not be a chore but a respectful choice*

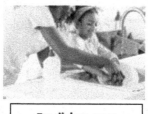

Do dishes, as a choice, not a chore

- Food is wasted in many homes, school cafeterias, or holiday parties. Will such wastage of resources be your bad karma, and will you be responsible for being a silent party to the collective wrongful act? **Answer is YES**

- The principle of not wasting food, energy, or time calms the head and enlarges the heart. Your intelligence (buddhi) is at work in making the right choices. Similar cosmic intelligence aka *mahat* is at work universally, including the routine act of eating. You are partaking cosmic intelligence by ingesting the grains. *Anna Hey Poorna Brahma* is a **Hindu prayer** at eating time.

*TIP: *Give respect to get respect* - this applies to living beings and things or objects.

ACT- 9: SLEEP WELL EVERY NIGHT

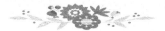

TIP 1: Sleep comes easy when you're breathing deep and rhythmic and when you've no objectives left to do during the day

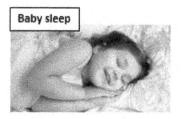

TIP 2: Treat **insomnia** like drug addiction; both are bad habits to be kicked out

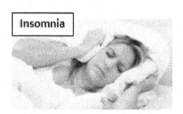

STEP 1: First Aid- Get to the root cause: Ex. Sleep posture, restless legs, caffeine drinks late at night, alcohol, painful joints, constipation, or poor breathing.

STEP 2: For curing Restless Legs Syndrome in the middle of the night: try slow Yogic walking for 5 min & Legs up wall pose, or with some pending work accomplished by the hands, such as Talasan pose, or writing a donation check.

STEP 3: Lying in bed on your back, do the following breathing kriyas

    i.   Consciously take stock of the accomplishments in the day while deep breathing

ii. also, hold breath 1 sec after inhaling, & watch stray thoughts, like clouds disappearing in the sky. Exhale with Root lock, and drift into Yog Nidra

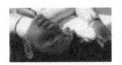

YOG nidra

STEP 4: Do a chair pose on a straight-backed chair, and legs uncrossed. After 2 – 3 deep breaths, let your eyes roll up to gaze at the third eye chakra # 6. Trick the mind by an imposed rhythm of the fingers patting. Repeat, keep track of musical breathing and patting till insomnia disappears

STEP 5: At bedtime, avoid: (i) ***Kapalbhati*** or a serious stretch (ii) an engaging TV show. Instead, take a warming bath (or soak feet in warm water), massage soles in sesame oil, and keep the cold towel on head

STEP 6: Consult your doctor if the above simple measures do not put you to sleep, and ask if any OTC (Over the Counter) pills containing herbs and natural ingredients may help as a sleep supplement.

Eating a compatible diet for easy digestion, doing Yog asanas (to improve posture), and sleeping 7- 8 hours (to undo daily wear and tear) boost your well-being.

My own experience is that insufficient hours of sleep mean a more incredible urge to eat a low-quality, fat-rich, high–carb diet. If uncontrolled, weight gain, obesity, diabetes, and constipation.

10 years ago, I used to brag about 4 hours of sleep foolishly. This is an example of wrong knowledge (called *Viparyaya* by Patanjali [YS I.8]

SIGNS OF SLEEP DEPRIVATION

Further, the people who slept 5 hours or less had an 82% higher risk of heart attack and 32% higher risk than those who slept only 6 hours. Heart attack is the # 1 killer in the USA, in seniors and adults 30 - 45 y/o.

Dozing off/yawning while driving, watching TV, reading, or sitting in meetings; memory issues; difficulty focusing, slower reaction time during driving, and negativity/depression prematurely. 55% of American adults suffer from sleep deprivation. It is becoming an epidemic.

MORE SLEEP TIPS:

- Sleep with the head pointing to the geographical South. (Avoid pointing to North)

- Begin sleeping on the left side/change side when awakening.

- Avoid sleeping on your stomach or your back for an extended time.

- Take a cupful of warm hot milk with ½ tsp of turmeric powder at bedtime.

- Do meditation on the floor or in bed.

- In my case, eating Vata balancing Dashmula or isabgol herb also helped.

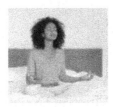

Meditate in Bed

ACT- 10: MANAGING EMOTION CURES DEPRESSION

Learn to honor breath-

The body gets fit,

The mind thinks better,

Heart becomes kinder

TWO HUMANS (ID=BODY/MIND/SPIRIT)

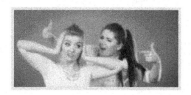   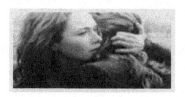

No Contact/

yet 'Ego tussle' & Long-term
dispute

Loving Contact/

No yelling, & dispute resolved

Follows complex energy exchange Law

Action can be feeling, thought, word or behavior

Reaction (return of energy) is more complex*

Maybe in this lifetime or in future lives

TWO OBJECTS (ID=SHAPE/SIZE)

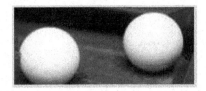   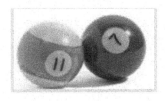

No Contact/	Yes Contact/
No action No reaction	**Equal, & Instant Reaction**

Follows simple physics law

Action/reaction: are measurable forces

Reaction (force) = Action simple & predictable

Must be now or soon

*Managing thoughts, moods, feelings, and sentiments blinds you as alcohol does, but the habit can alter by training in yoga.

TIP: It is practical to teach breathing in school and the Laws of Physics.

Society will benefit- How not harm yourself or release adrenaline or cortisol in public?

Three controllable Emotions: Anger, Delusion, Fear

Hasty Reaction is wrong/Reasoned Response for every mood is right

A hasty reaction means punishing yourself for the wrongs committed by some other

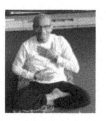

Supt-padmasan

Freedom from Fear, Anger and Delusion is crucial to preserve the yogic gains from Asana/Pranayama.

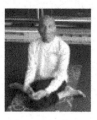

Pranayama P4

Fear means an injustice may occur, and your instant hasty reaction is out of frustration. Will this wrong happen to me?

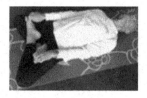

Gomukhasan

The dilemma – either repression (bottling up the anger, hiding the emotion, such as pressure in a closed soda water bottle), or expression (letting it out in a fury, displaying in screaming or hollering, like spraying soda on the opponent's face) The healthy response to anger.

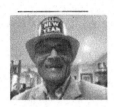

Muktahaas (laugh)pose

There is a third and simpler alternative to knock anger out of your system: by understanding the very roots of anger, the knack of watching. Close your eyes, breathe deep, search, and find there was no root cause other than your habitual lifestyle. The harmful emotion would not recur in the future. (In teaching STEM courses in the colleges, the common advice is: 'Read the question paper for 10 minutes to plan the strategy.'

Yoga postures to control Anger include the Sun Salutation

TIP: Deep breathe + Understand + Analyze = Tame the mind

DEPRESSION/ANXIETY

The mind, usually the boss, behaves like a slave*.

- Depression is a disorderly mood, anxiety, or emotion, and interferes with a person's ability to work, sleep, study, eat and enjoy.

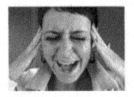

  - One every 40 seconds, that's how often, according to WHO- people die by suicide, and it adds up to nearly 800,000 people globally every year, incl school kids. It's estimated that 60% of those committing suicide are plagued by major depression.

  - A report by Blue Cross Blue Shield found that depression in the US alone has risen dramatically after the 'stay at home' orders. Current psychiatric drugs have failed to curtail this growing crisis, with dangerous side effects and losing 100s of billion dollars in earnings per year.

- The good news! Choose an act which you can do better now than before Ex. P1- P4 *pranayam*, followed by low impact, gentle poses- Child pose, *Viprit-karni*, *Savasan* helps in building self-defense, with lesser Rx use.

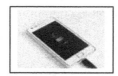

- Slower breathing and mindfulness cool down the sympathetic nervous system, adding anti-bodies, and preventing the spread of infection in the corona virus.

- One domestic remedy is drinking herbal tea made of ¼ teaspoon of holy basil and ½ teaspoon of sage per cup of hot water twice a day or more, instead of drinking alcohol or soda.

- Rubbing the top of the head and soles of the feet with sesame oil is soothing for vata depression. (Vata is a characteristic dosha of many seniors). However, your Ayurvedic medics need to be checked by a trained practitioner, who may prescribe proven natural herbs with no side effects

- As general health improves, memory returns and the 'enslaved mind' remembers its superior authority and trains the line managers to stay within their assigned roles—order returns. Depression ends.

Practical applications

In social/political life, it is right to stand tall, confident, looking up, then you do not allow anyone to offend you or your country.

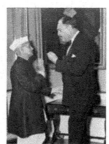

**L. B. Sastry on left
& Ayub Khan**

The picture shows the small frame of Indian Prime Minister Lal Bahadur Shastry facing the tall Pakistani Pres. Ayub Khan in Tashkent, USSR (now Uzbekistan) in 1966.

- A reporter asked a demeaning question, and P.M. Shastry un-nerved the opponent, 'I am looking up, confident, Mr. Khan is looking down, dejected.'

- If you feel inferior and get upset- you are punishing yourself and snapping the connection with the divinity within you. This is insane!

- Every morning, thank heavens for being alive and remind yourself to work with noble intent and sincere effort, and the day turns in your favor.

- With gratitude to yourself, & God on your side, other smart acts shall follow.

I've read a book: 'Good things happen to Good people'- This may be absurd, but it is an unfailing justice.

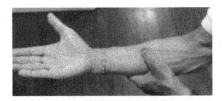

Life battery charging

• **TIP:** To keep the life battery charged on the go, apply acupressure treatment daily on the right hand between the wrist and the elbow.

Two minutes of acupressure every morning maintains youthfulness in the day and keeps the mind refreshed as long as you live.

A refreshed mind is not a devil's workshop.

Lastly, consider yoga as a Satsang between man and the divine. Learn how to be a better yogi.

ACT- 11: YOUR RIGHTS TO REDEEM

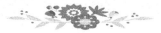

Whatever you do, think, or say, you are doing a karmic act. Yogi, however, consciously makes it good karma. Also,

1. **Right to make choices-** As a practicing yogi, you'd realize it is your fundamental right to you, and assist others to do so, be it a living being or non-living object. Moreover, when choosing between the good/evil, profit/loss, now or later, try 10 minutes of your favorite asana/pranayama, and wow, you get a clearer vision and direction. This may be so because humans can stand, balanced, in equilibrium on two feet only.

2. **Right to thrive.** Let us hope the teaching in school or college goes beyond how to invest in 401K. Teaching must also include how to thrive in golden years. Then, the seniors don't suffer from chronic illnesses, are forced to live secluded in long-term care, or die untimely.

3. **Right to be knowledgeable-** Unfortunately, many seniors may be wondering why they were ignorant of yoga or the difference between information and knowledge. The State Law gives you the "Right to Information (RTI)" but not the "Right to Knowledge (RTK)." Six months before retiring, why not make RTK a mandatory benefit, and then most seniors will practice yoga.

4. **Right to be rewarded-** It is also your Right to be aware that you were born with genes of meditation and not to forget that you were a child-yogi. This awareness will let you live healthy till the last breath. When the time is ripe, you will die singing God's glory. Friends and family will celebrate such death and be inspired by your living example. Can there be a better redemption?

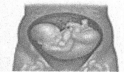
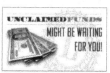

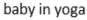
baby in yoga
Embryo in meditation
Forgotten treasure
(similar to inner soul)

So, two points- i) choose to be knowledgeable and ii) redeem the rewards on the go.

ACT- 12: MEDITATE DAILY

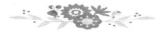

Sleep relaxes the body; Meditation relaxes the Mind

Even 10-minutes can be a Daily tonic

 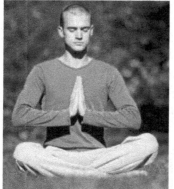 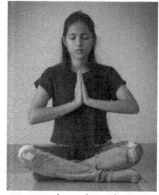

Conscious namaste pose   un-conscious drooping arm

A short poem!

Whenever lonesome or bereft, I sit down spine, & head Erect

Close my eyes, Lips in Smile, Practice Nadi Shodhan for a while

Chant Sohum, inhaling 'so', exhaling 'hum'

Five senses perceive: hear, smell, think, taste, or see

There is peace and light inside, Is it Ajnya chakra in Sight

Simply happening, or spiritual awakening

I open my Eyes, ten gates I count, but see nothing moving in or out.

What is and what is not Meditation?

- Everyone wants to cultivate a happy attitude within & gain external happiness. Meditation does both.

- Meditation is discovery of your real nature sat, chit, Anand, and is beyond intellectual reasoning. Knowing that your essence is consciousness is Bliss.

- It is the unbroken awareness of Truth for a minimum of 20 minutes, without interruption.

- It is the state of Being and transforming slothful and egotistical tendencies of the human mind.

Pre-requisites of meditation- make it your daily discipline (dharma)

- Cleansing yourself inside/out is the initial step (yam/niyam)

- For steady posture, sit upright, aligned, and comfortable on the ground (Asana)

- For rhythmic breathing, do four basic kriyas

- For senses withdrawal, do Bhramari pranayama and Yoni mudra (pratyahar)

- For true concentration, do advanced mudras (dharna)

- Now, you are meditation-worthy, i.e., ready to meditate (dhyan)

How Long to meditate?

-Start with 2 minutes of deep breathing- long inhale and stepwise filling the lungs with oxygen & extended exhale, pushing the toxins out of the body. Slowly you're drifting to a higher state of consciousness.

After that, time flies as you 'taste' bliss, experience light without a visible source, patience, tapas, and the virtues of your choice follow!

-Remember, the ultimate goal is the self-awakening you have been waiting for, then grace gur prasad fills up the empty spot in your heart.

Conclusion

- Meditation can be the most proficient technique to harness energy.

- For retired seniors, it is fun to practice meditation in action.

- Ward off stray thoughts by chanting your ishta mantra.

Dalai Lama in meditation for long hours

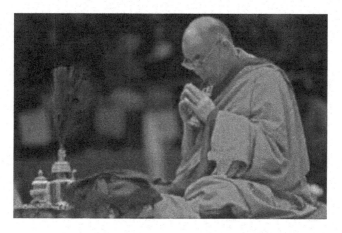

Five methods of Meditation-choose what suits you best.

Firstly, you must know yourself and your tendencies/habits- the good and not so good.

1. **AUM meditation** – For a higher connection

   - Aum is the auspicious universal sound and has multiple meanings. Most significant is its three sounds, A, U, M, ending in silence.

   - AUM conveys Consciousness underlying 3 states - waking, sleeping, dreamless sleep, and the silence at the end.

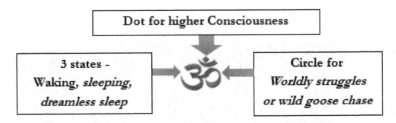

Dot for higher Consciousness

| 3 states – Waking, *sleeping, dreamless sleep* | | Circle for *Worldly struggles or wild goose chase* |

   - Another meaning is Consciousness of the human effort of three entities body/mind/intellect.

   - Inhale in 3 sec/exhale 3 sounds and the silence each 3 sec (total 15 sec), followed by brief *mulbandh kriya*.

   - You would feel freshness manifesting in the body, fluctuations of mind ceasing, and AUM in the crown.

2. **Sohum meditation**

   - This practice yokes the individual with the universal cosmic consciousness.

   - On inhalation, mentally chant 'so' (pronounced Sah), gazing tip of your nose.

   - On exhalation, resonate the sound Hum. Listen to the Sohum sound in the whole breath, and visualize your breathing is becoming quieter and spontaneous

- For the timed meditation option, inhale/exhale needs to be equal, inhale in long O combining A and U sounds, and exhale in long M....non-stop. Repeat for the set time of meditation.

3. Five Senses meditation: for Progressive Relaxation

Once you have enjoyed the calming effect, you can advance to 5-senses meditation.

Open your mouth slightly, and your tongue touches the roof of the mouth, behind the upper teeth.

Begin by paying attention to the sense of inner hearing, the feeble, and the loud notes for 1-2 minutes.

Then pay attention to the senses of inner vision, followed by smell, taste, and touch.

Explore which sense gives better calmness for a total of 10 – 20 min.

4. Third eye meditation: For clarity

Close the eyes, with gaze turned up between the eyebrows, you may experience queer pleasantness in the forehead, a luminous shine at or near the third eye. An after-effect is- to combine a spiritual orientation with daily activities to work without fatigue during the day and sleep better at night.

5. Insight meditation – for an extended duration

Choose an object for gazing that is interesting and meaningful such as a flower, Aum symbol, or a moorthy kept at eye level. Do mantra jap with sustained rhythmic breathing.

You will feel a mystery doorway opening inside the closed eyes, without any fixed identity.

- Do not terminate the meditation in a hurry. Rub your hands and let the pleasing warmth flow gently to your eyes and senses. Then slowly open your eyes.

- Mindfully, sing a prayer and get up slowly, exchanging Namaste with all present. Then, you establish a sacred binding connection with members of the group!

    i) In meditation, it is OK to be alone (ekant), to rejoice you are on your journey.

    ii) When alone, first make friends with your senses and body organs; they must feel cared.

iii) For example- meditating on your spine can ease back pain. Child pose makes you humble.

iv) Opportunities for innovation- exploring the unknown- are many.

v) A sample of easy breathing meditation follows

TIP: Meditation should initially be practiced for 10 minutes, raising it by a minute or two every week to 30 minutes.

4 easy steps: 1. Sit correctly 2. Watch breath 3. Wait to be quiet 4. Witness the mind, no judging

MEDITATION IS NOW GLOBALLY PRACTICED

8 Steps to make a beginning today

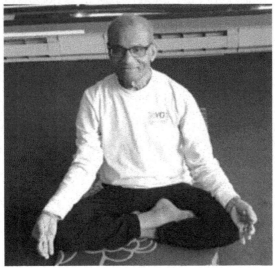

Gyan mudra

1. **Place & Time:** Find 15 minutes in a noise-free place.

2. **Sit** facing east with the un-perturbed mind in a posture as shown, or sit in a chair.

    -   **Keep your** spine, head, and neck aligned; eyes semi-open, gently gazing at the tip of the nose to avoid eye strain.

    -   **Keep hands** on thighs in any of the two mudras shown or the mudra of choice to assist in contemplation.

3. **Breathing.** Do P4 Pranayama, or just breathe thru the nose slow, rhythmic, inhale/ exhale of equal duration 3 sec each. Repeat 3 cycles.

4. **Scan:** Starting from the toes, mentally scan your body, moving up toward the legs, torso, neck, and head.

    -   Visualize cool energy flowing in your nostrils, inhaling and warm toxins, & anxiety flowing out in exhaling.

    -   Now you're getting meditation ready.

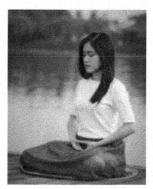

Buddha mudra

5. **Concentrate.** Continue gazing on the tip of your nose, or any object kept at eye level will do.

    Chant the 'So-hum' mantra, and imagine the object's halo as eyes go self-shut.

6. **Be aware** of your ongoing deep breathing, Inhale 'So'/Exhale 'Hum,' experiencing peace and calm, as you can refocus from distractions.

7. **Gratitude.** After the set time, rub both palms and gently place warm palms on closed eyes, then on the forehead, nose, ears, face, neck, and the medulla plexus on the back of the head.

8. **End.** Conclude by mental chanting of

    Tamaso Ma Jyotirgamaya,

    Asato Ma Satgamaya,

    Mrityorma Amritam Gamaya.

Open your eyes. Smile and bow down to all present.

Now you're ready to face life with greater confidence and less fear.

CONCLUSION: PART ONE

Yoga is the science of healthy living for all

- Three types of people usually practice yoga

i) A healthy person wants to remain socially active for life- basic 20-min daily yoga is their goal.

A few of them with higher aim do advanced yoga plus 30- min or more of meditation.

ii) A sick person If diagnosed with a health issue- yoga 'Nips the Evil in the Bud,' and helps revert to healthy person status i)- if yoga becomes their new lifestyle.

iii) A sick person If diagnosed with chronic illness (diabetes, BP, cardio, cancer, domestic violence, depression), yoga may prevent it from worsening further, and live in a peace in-home setting.

- Follow your favorite leaders Ex. **Narendra Modi** of India, and **Abe Lincoln** of the USA.

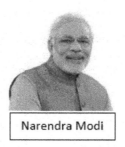

Narendra Modi

They rose from humble beginnings, set goals, achieved higher objective, and others got inspired.

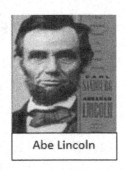

Abe Lincoln

Such leaders come on planet earth for a specific purpose and time. They would physically pass, but their memory lives forever. Selfless action is their noble aim!

Yoga is India's major contribution to the world because no one is ever too weak- physically or mentally-as not to do light yoga, breathe, pray, meditate and chant.

- The future of therapy must be the union of traditional yoga and modern medicine.

- A message is seen on WhatsApp- 'At the individual level, bath purifies the body, breath purifies the mind, and yoga purifies the whole body/mind and spirit.

4-types of devotees: Afflicted (arta), Inquisitive (jigyasu), Needy (arthi), Savant (gyani)

PM Modi, yogi-cum-politician believes in peace yet speaks the language of surgical Strike when dealing with terrorists.

PART TWO:

WHY DO YOGA?

22-TOPICS ON SWADHYAYA FOR STUDY OF SELF SVATMA

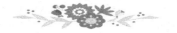

Einstein said- 'Science without Religion is Lame.'

Lord Krishna of India proclaimed 5000 years ago

'Action(abhyas) without intention (Sankalp),

Wealth(dhan) without wisdom(buddhi) is also Lame.'

Therefore, Hindus often worship twin gods at Diwali time-Lakshmi, the goddess of wealth, and Ganesh, the god of wisdom.

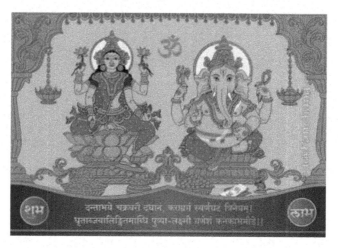

The two gods are inseparable* for true success

*More inseparable- Arjuna & Krishna (Nar & Narayan) + ve pride svabhiman & sub-conscious mind

body/mind with higher power transcend raw brain & partner with intellect

Similarly, saint Tulsi Das wrote in Ramayana, describing the two kinds of inseparable-sumati (goodwill) & sampati(wealth) are +ve inseparable, as the body/mind are trained to cooperate

Jahan Sumati, Tahan Sampati Nana - where is goodwill, affection, friendly attitude, there is wealth, prosperity, victory, and wellness

Jahan Kumati, Tahan Vipati Nidana - Jahan Kumati, Tahan Vipati Nidana, there is poverty, trouble, defeat, and illness

In the English language, it goes- **'Misfortunes never come alone.'**

Hence, be cautious to Nip the evil in the bud. Else a molehill becomes a mountain, or a minor illness becomes chronic.

1. WHY CHOOSE YOG PLUS GYM

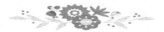

- **What is Yoga and what is not Yoga?**

  - Yoga is your base existence; you feel a void and loss of direction without it.

  - The short-term goal of many is to get rid of the Rx pills and create conditions to improve the survival level.

  - **Yoga is to** experience the inner treasure behind the stillness of mind and closed eyes. You get vitality in body and mind with yoga- you are now at the higher level, aka yogic union.

  - Creating conditions of a yogic union, similar to the nuclear fusion of Helium nuclides, is your responsibility. But doing nothing or waiting for the magic to happen randomly is incapable *ayogya*.

  - Yoga is knowing what is meaningful to do and not succumbing to the temptation of what is not right.

  - As advocated in the eBook, YOG starts with purifying the body, mind, and heart, aka shauch.

  - Although a very old Indian tradition, Yoga is universal and continues to appeal in modern times.

  - YOG is fun + intelligent; its gains are far-reaching,

    curing sleeping disorders, high/low BP, anxiety/stress, obesity, diabetes, cancer, and heart ailments.

- **Many yoga options** are described in PART TWO of the Book.

  - There is no age bar: yoga is compatible with seniors, children, office workers, or retirees.

  - Yoga is an added weapon to fight infection and build immunity, with few side effects.

  - Criminals in jail can be rehabilitated and their behavior transformed as responsible citizens.

- A digitized treadmill displays the expected outcome in real-time.

- The same is true if you wear a smart Apple watch for on-go feedback and inspiration.

Ultimately, in the 21st century, the popular health slogan must be **Let Yog & Gym unite.**

2. FOUR GREAT QUESTIONS (MAHAVAKYAS)

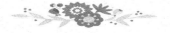

Who Am I? Whence have I come? Why have I come? Where will I go?

- **These questions** reflect the higher knowledge described in the wisdom book, Kathopanishad, as a dialog between the young seeker Nachiketa and Yama, the Lord of Death. Nachiketa requested Yama to reveal the secret knowledge of Death. Yama tried to test the boy before revealing.

- **Upanishads** preach: You have a material body, which is mortal; it is born, grows, decays, and dies. You also have an immortal Being- the soul/spirit Consciousness

The soul is shrouded, like an herbal tea bag whose aroma is locked inside the paper. Make use of the yogic knowledge to relax instead of running around aimlessly. Ex. Two birds in a tree. The higher relaxed bird, having gained knowledge, is relaxed. The lower bird, wayward mind, keeps running and finally misses the goal.

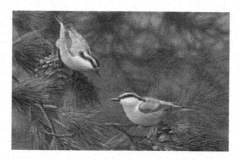

- Karma- a compulsive bodily deed, spoken word, or a created emotion. *Karmas* are of 3 types-

   i) *(sanchit)* the net tally of accumulated karmas from previous births,

   ii) *(prarabdh)* part of sanchit karma allocated to be executed in the present life,

iii) (*kriyaman*) the portion or all of prarabdh being finished in the present life.

Note: the unfinished prarabdh goes back to the sanchit pool.

- To most people, *karma* appears to be perpetual bondage. But by handling your allotted act responsibly, *karma* can be the stepping stone to final liberation. This means fewer cases of untimely death, chronic sickness or depression, or lack of devotion midway. In other words, one may not always choose the task, but the skill of completing it smartly is certainly an option. Yoga is knowing the difference *karma vs. karmayoga?*

TIP: When acting consciously, you'd become aware that heaven or hell is not geographical place but a quality of the process– how well the task is completed.

3. SANKHYA YOG...AT A GLANCE

All body parts are assigned individual as well as collective goals*

25 QUALITY ELEMENTS	Inter dependence	21 BODY PARTS	
1-5: Five gross Elements - (Mahabhutas - Earth, Water, Fire, Air, and Ether)		21	Head
		20	Neck
6-9: Four Internal equipment- (antahkaran) Mind- Sensory-motor mind (Manas) Intellect - Discriminative faculty (Buddhi) Ego - Fake Individuality (Ahamkar) Consciousness - (chitta)		19	Back
		18	Shoulder
		16, 17	Arm
		15	Hand
10-19: Ten external equipment- (Bahyakaran) 5 senses of Cognition (Gyanendriyas) - seeing, smelling, hearing, taste, touch) 5 senses of Action (Karmendriyas) - Hands, Feet, Mouth, gates of elimination)		13, 14	Wrist, elbow
		11, 12	Fingers, thumb
		9, 10	Hip, belly
20. Material equipment- Prakruti (Maya)	Tadasana - a pose for body- care	7, 8	Knee, Thigh
		5, 6	Ankle, Calf
21-25: Five subtle elements (Tanmatras) - form, odor, sound, flavor, contact)		3, 4	Big, small toes
		1, 2	Foot, heel/sole

* Thru simple 'tense release' method, each body part stays healthy, increasing your life span.

- It is your responsibility to raise each body part lovingly, like massaging your baby.

- Feeding with love into your heart will last longer; feeding with jealousy ends in a heart attack.

TIP: Your mouth and mind- the tongue and the ego- can be your best friend or enemy.

21 body parts

Arm- 8 pairs
(Finger, thumb, wrist, elbow, hand, fore arm, upper arm, shoulder)
Leg-8 pairs
(Foot, toe, ankle, calf, knee, leg, thigh, butt)
Belly-1
Back*-1
Neck-1
Chest-1
Head-1

*There is no joint in the back bone; so, a healthy back is flat, hunch-free

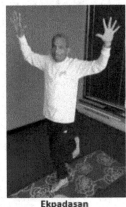

Ekpadasan

6 SENSES

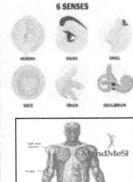

6 major joints

- Sufferings are usually of 3-kinds (trividha), and these are a consequence of karma in the past

  i) (*Daihik*)- from your wrongdoing- resulting in a sick body and/or a foggy mind.

    The good news is these ills are treatable/preventable by timely diagnosis and yogic kriyas.

  ii) (*Bhautik*)- from other earthly beings- neighbors, insect bites, animal attacks, rape of women, etc.

    Social laws, community involvement, and insurance protection do help.

  iii) (*Daivik*)- from unearthly acts- tremors, tsunamis, floods, pandemics, wildfires, aka the act of God.

    Community yagnas, divine intervention, training camps, and protocol guidelines help.

Likewise, sufferings are healed by removing the cause of ignorance (ajnan), lack of vitality (ashakt), lack of resources (abhav). The eBook provides instructions for help

- To love your spouse is your karma. To love yourself is your dharma. Then Your conduct (acharan) with family and friends improves, and goodwill grows within and around you.

- By the Law of Attraction, a healthy body adjusts according to the dictates of the subconscious. The seven good habits are formed through the four interlinked areas of self-care.

- **The sixth sense of** Intuition develops as ignorance-driven limitations are removed. This is your 'right to knowledge'

TIP: In an Asana pose, when you're unable to stretch enough, it is OK to hold midway, close the eyes, inhale and affirm as if additional healing energy has been dispatched to that body part.

Injury is real, but pain/suffering is mental and preventable with the right attitude.

Material success in the world may dictate pressure and stress, but emotional maturity brings calm without fear, anxiety, or tension now or later.

Hence the need for yoga to balance the two opposites and make life a whole-hearted involvement.

You can control early aging and the untimely death-

I love my new SUV car; its sensory cameras and ongoing input signals, an imaginary surround sound (a virtual dummy is in the passenger seat), keep offering a friendly warning of traffic ahead, incl. A cop in hiding- is it 6th sense?

Virtual-dummy

Imagine yourself on life's superhighway and manifesting greater youthful energy and meaning in life.

The yogic lifestyle in vanprastha retirement stage when run without bitterness, frustration, or anger. may add up to 7 years to a healthy lifespan.

The basic pranayamas and Suryanamaskar chair poses, as described in p. 124-125, must be studied before retiring. Then the treasure of retired life reveals to make you feel richer than you had ever imagined.

It can be appreciated why yogis are less likely to fall sick or suffer to the same degree as couch-potato seniors? Also, a yogi by creative inquiry, safe stretching at a higher-level recover faster from an unexpected sickness?

A yogi learns to guard against early aging by i) daily +ve yoga, ii) eating fresh with low tamasic content, iii) breathing deep, and iv) 3Rs.

A yogi's body, mind, and heart age at the same rate, then he dies fearless like a ripened cucumber falling from the vine, as described in the Mahamrityunjaya mantra. Sickness becomes a stepping stone!

In social meetings, the usual question is, 'Ravi ji, at what age did you Yog'? My humble reply with a twist is 'when I was eight years older.

Yoga has been my re-birth, as these recent years are adding years. I feel the pinch if I do not do daily yoga!

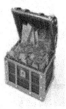

Forgotten treasure- a gift of old age

TIP: 'YOG well, eat sensibly, and you'll be happy like never before.

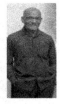

Author
86 y/o

4. FIVE BODIES TO THE SELF (*PANCH KOSH/LAYERS*)

Accessing the 5 layers in sequence leads to divine spiritual knowledge

- The resident- **jivatma** in the human body, is surrounded by five layers, bodies, koshas, or sheaths. For the outermost physical layer 1, food (*anna*) is necessary for survival. Layer 2, the breath body *pranomay* kosh directly regulates lower intelligence aka *manomaya* kosh layer 3, mostly -ve ego. *Vignanmaya kosh,* the emotional body layer 4 opens the door to higher intelligence and +ve ego. One who understands its functioning modulates his reactions, emotions, urges, and temptations, leading to purposeful life sooner or later.

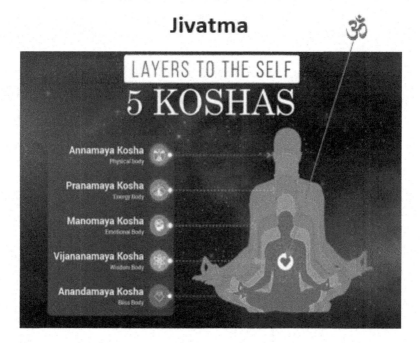

- • Doing yogic practice from an early age, you're capable to grasp the futility of getting stuck at layers 1,2,3; this is true for only 4% people. They ultimately reach at layer 4, a step away from the inner Bliss body 5*

- • The multi-layer concept is utilized as 'defense in depth' in the most modern nuclear power plants for robust design, quality construction, trained operation/maintenance crew, security, and planned containment of accidents.

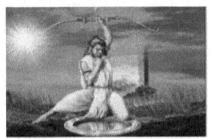

Arjuna, hero of Mahabharat pierced the fish eye, as Krishna stilled the water pond.

* Note: At Layer 5, the yogi has attained, yet she may or may not leave the world like a siddha yogi like Buddha.

Shai Weiss, CEO of Virgin Atlantic, said in a recent 40-sec speech, 'Finish office work in time, come home in time. He meant to balance home & office.

Aim: physically healthy aka survive mode			Aim: Meaningful life aka thrive mode		
LAYER 1	**LAYER 2**	**LAYER 3**	**LAYER 4**	**LAYER 5**	**KEY**
Annamay kosha	Pranamay kosha	Manomay kosha	Vijnanmay kosha	Anandmay kosha	Sanskrit name
Physical/ Gross body (outermost)	Pranic/ Energy/ breath body	Mental/ Thinking body	Emotional body sadbuddhi	Spiritual body (innermost)	Common name
Ache-free body	Common name	-ve Ego joins lower intelligence	+ve Ego joins higher intelligence	Mental Peace	Initial gain
Stability	Vitality Better breathing	Success	Wisdom	Experience the wow!	Potential gain

Asana	Pranayama	Pre-meditation (mindfulness)	Meditation	More meditation	Recommended yoga step
				◄	

TIP:

1. The usual human sufferings- muscular aches, pains, mental stress, anxiety, worry, bad mood, and obesity, ups and downs govern – the root cause is not doing right asanas/kriyas.

2. When you do the sadhana under the guidance of a teacher, layers 1, 2, and 3 are brought into alignment, and more room is created effortlessly for higher awareness to blossom.

3. Layers 4 and 5 become self-activated, which leads to self-transformation.

5. ETERNAL LAWS/TRUTHS OF NATURE

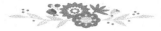

The world is governed by eternal laws which keep unfolding like a flower.

The choice to follow or ignore the Laws is yours; you must bear the consequences.

- Some of the eternal Laws are listed below.

    - Law of Action: Doing an act leads to understanding and turns knowledge into wisdom

    - Law of Unity: You may be separate beings and destinies, yet connected to one Truth

    - Law of Balance: Find the mid-way in whatever you do, think or feel

    - Law of Choices: You may not control a circumstance but can choose your response

    - Law of Integrity: Live up to your vision, despite impulses to the contrary

    - Law of Presence: Realize the power of each moment; time is a social convenience

    - Law of Process: A big journey can be transformed into a series of small steps

    - Law of Deserving: Nature provides what you deserve, not what you desire. Ex. In a job interview, you are hired if your qualifications primarily meet the employer's needs, and you may have to adjust to enhance the expectations.

- Three acts enhance deserving notes 1, and 2 and allow grace to enter your life: Keep the divine pot (i) open/upright, (ii) clean, and (iii) leak-free. This is also the message in 5 Layers; when layers 1, 2, and 3 are aligned you become deserving.

Divine Grace

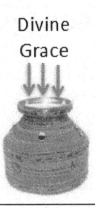

> **Carry the pot, charged like the cell phone**

Remember, insurance payment kicks in after you've made the co-payment.

Note 1: At birth, God gifts everyone with body, mind, intelligence, and a pot to top it with divine grace.

Note 2: Understand the difference between the divine eternal Laws and artificial dogmas

More laws govern during life in this and in that world-

Law of Evolution: Without passion, there is no evolution or happiness

Law of Freewill: Law of freedom to choose to evolve or not

Law of justice, cause/effect: Law of physical and spiritual action/reaction

Ex.1:   Exhale is as important as inhale

Ex.2:   Remove weeds before sowing seeds

Ex.3:   Relax well to work hard

Ex.4:   Spending well is as important as earning

Ex.5:   There is social justice improving the life of people, such as abolishing slavery, triple talaq, and more

Caution: An unwritten eternal law is 'self-regulation.' Who reminds earth of the gravitational pull? A human, however, needs a constant reminder...

Suggestion: Let your child put a dollar in the box for each deviation! There would be enough money to start a new business someday!

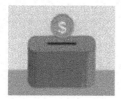

Doing *sattvic* duties are your primary rights- to transcend the limitations Make peace, health, and happiness your acts of worship- so says Sri Sri Ravi Shankar.

* Eternal Laws are a joint venture between humans and the divine. That is why the principle- Man proposes/God disposes of. This includes your daily work impacting not only the individual but also social and cosmic good. That defines a weak-willed or a strong-willed community!

6. YOUR SPIRITUAL METER

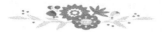

The spiritual highway displays good omens

- Life is often messy. Ex. poison and nectar co-existed in the mythical ocean churning.

Arjuna, the skilled warrior of the Mahabharata war, chose Krishna to be his guide/friend and control the 4 white horses (symbolic of dynamism and devotion). If their reins (symbolic of mental functions) are controlled, else horses will go astray if the reins are not tightened properly.

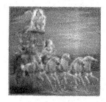

Typical symptoms/omens of awakened Consciousness are the followings-

Yama & Niyama of yoga are commands of nature:	Yoga is becoming as important as air and water
Your annual wellness report is getting better:	Not blaming fate or DNA for your health problem
Deep breathing and healing are inter-related, similar to right intention, posture, and back pain:	Timely check-ups can prevent chronic illness.

Before eating, inquire if the meal is nutritious, to the yardsticks for a healthy body/mind/spirit?	Selfcare means controlling 'meaningless' desires, impulses, *vasanas,* and urges
Enjoy helping others in selfless ways:	Embrace 3R's on and off the yoga mat
Prioritize meditation, improved memory, and root cause analysis...are means to know God:	Friends dis-agree, yet hold hands & move forward; a dying soldier wishes recovery to other soldiers.
God gives material, and making the finished product is human effort.	Keep learning new skills, and life will be enriched

7. FOUR PILLARS (PURUSHARTHAS)

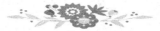

Moksha, ultimate Aim is realized when the three gunas have fulfilled their higher purpose

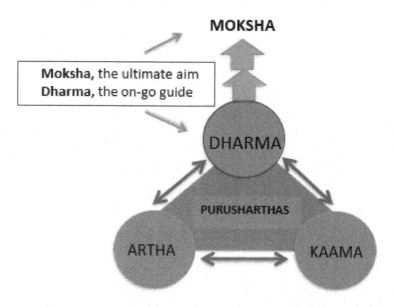

PURUSHARTHA: Four aims of life are:

    i)   **DHARMA** (Devout life) - Laws that uphold righteousness

    ii)   **ARTHA** (Material pursuit)[1] - Make a living that pays bills

    iii) **KAAMA** (Pleasure pursuit)[1] - Sensuous enjoyments

    iv) **MOKSHA** (Spiritual pursuit) - Ultimate beatitude

[1] Partly destiny from the past lives

In summarizing, the actions of artha and kaama need to be performed with the guidance of dharma to help the human race grow. It would be wrong to treat life like a trip to a gambling casino, where Dharma and Moksha are side lined.

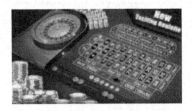

- Earth, since its formation more than 4.32 billion years ago, has been associated with twin motions

  i) rotates on its axis @ 1037 mph (15 naut-mile/min) speed at the equator to make day and night in a 24-hour cycle. Surprisingly, 15 bpm is the breathing rate of a normal healthy person.

  ii) races/revolves around the sun @ 67,000 mph (30 km/sec), to make seasons in 365.25 days cycle.

  Moon orbits earth in a month (average 1 km/sec). From the above, you learn more about Eternal laws, namely

  a) It does not speed that kills; it is the acceleration, the emotional upheaval, the uncontrolled reaction.

  b) Laws of Presence and Balance define a relation between man and nature. Learn these.

- Honouring eternal laws, distinct from narrow-minded religions, dogmas, and traditions can

  - reform the outdated belief patterns. Ex. Triple Talaq was declared illegal in India

  - religious leaders, and politicians need to accept the simplification of other outdated customs which violate the changing social aspirations of today's citizens.

- BG Ch. 10, Sh. 4, 5 describe 20 feelings; only four arise from God's impulsion*, and the rest are self-created from motivated actions of the individual. Hence, controllable....

- Modern sages Baba Ramdev, Sri Ravi Shanker & Sadhguru Vasudev, are going the extra mile to popularize Yoga beyond declaring June 21 the International Day of Yoga.

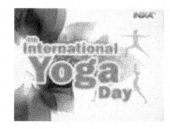

A suggestion- It would be worthwhile to award a penalty of 1-week compulsory YOG practice to an erring driver jumping a red light, to discipline a roadside vendor for not disposing of the garbage, or to a student for not completing the homework on time.

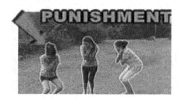

Similarly, God will put you to the austerity test if you are worthy of learning a lesson.

Negative ego changes to positive humility, and you're gaining physical as well as mental health, accepting the karmas with grace

---

*Birth/death, fame/infamy, happiness/unhappiness, fear/fearlessness are divine gifts; God sends opportunity at an appropriate time when you are ready to face a challenge.

8. SAMSKARAS ARE FORMED 4 WAYS

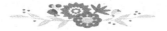

- An intent thought or act leaves its imprint on the mind, and these become your deep-rooted tendencies, aka samskara, a Sanskrit term (Sam means planned, kara means action).

- Samskaras impel a man for more desires and actions and are planted 4 ways in our body (1).

  i) Genes: what you carry forward from this or previous lives– ex. physical look, special talent, or hereditary trait (obesity, cancer, diabetes, temperament and/or perceptions)

  ii) Upbringing: what you acquire from parents' habits, religious leaning, values, and rituals at home.

  iii) Learning: what you learn in school, peers, teachers, colleagues, travel, & self-study (2)

  iv) Spirituality: the permanence of the Soul/Spirit, the Realism, the Sat in you that make your heartbeat, blood flow, and wisdom grow. This is your permanent identity, the imperishable Chaitanya atma (3)

- Research proves that raising a child from conception to 5 years of age contributes significantly to their growth. Parents need to be careful that the child does not imbibe incorrect behavior later in life, such as chronic poor nutrition, bad temper, and anger/anxiety-like a termite silently eating into the foundation logs of the house.

- Furthermore, your 'out-of-box' thinking (2), experiences, and efforts, backed by spiritual strength, can put tremendous power in your hands. Due to years of 'dust on the mirror,' consciousness may become covered in ignorance. Still, it can be revived and overcome the bondage of karma or desire with the right effort—for example, the illiterate highway robber who had changed to sage Valmiki, author of the Ramayana epic.

(1) Through Technology + YOG, you can eliminate many obstacles, incl. Genetic influences. Iyengar BKS (ref. 1) rightly defines good Samskara – freeing yourself from unjustified habits

(2) A friend's misbehaviour unto you reflects on his poor samskaras. On your part, stay calm and patiently arrive at the right solution rather than react angrily in a hurry. Practice builds upon good samskaras.

(3) 'Not to ignore the yogic Hindu traditions of India' was the prophetic call of Swami Vivekananda 130 years ago to free India out of centuries of poverty & misery. And BG 18.66- sarva dharman parityajya………

9. MINDFULNESS VS. MEDITATION

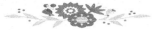

The supremacy of the human Mind has been recognized since ancient times.

I. Egyptian Sphinx and II. Ganesh, the Indian god of wisdom

- Meditation is understood as sitting steadily in a specific posture for a specific time. With eyes closed and mind turning inward – it is a journey from confused, fickle mind to attentive, no-mind.

- On the other hand, mindfulness directs your attention to the present act, whether sitting, talking, eating, shopping, or sleeping, as you are aware of the 3Rs.

- Ex.1: If you are sitting in a chair in an office meeting and adjusting your posture for the better, you are becoming more mindful. Or, if you practice Nishpandbhav , and yoni mudra

  - Ex.2: If you carefully analyze that your moves and urges are not disturbing other people in the neighborhood, you are also gaining in mindfulness.

  - Mindfulness is the practical handling of one bit at a time of a complex task if posture and breath be kept right. It can play the role of a trained assistant in the doctor's office when the doctor is busy.

  - People suffering from chronic pain, depression, and cancer have benefited from mindfulness combined with meditation. Here is a true story.

  - A patient on recognizing signs of depression, committed to being proactive, started doing specific yoga and ate nutritious meals. At times, she practiced psychotherapy for integrated well-being. She made a conscious effort to breathe deep and experience the pain as it was happening. She looked into the "pain's eye." The pain silently moved out thru her. She had developed the bad habit of building pressure to solve the problem.

- A similar strategy works for treating insomnia. I wear a pendant with 🕉 & Ganesh, the higher power protecting me as I tense and relax one body part at a time-toe to head.

10. AHAR, VIHAR, ACHAR, VICHAR - DYNAMIC LIFESTYLE

Inspired by a mural at The Yoga Institute, Mumbai, India

◄────── OUTER WORLD ──────►◄────── INNER WORLD ──────►			
I. *Ahar* ◄──► (Food/diet)	II. *Vihar* ◄──► (Relax/recharge)	III. *Achar* ◄──► (Code of conduct)	IV. *Vichar* (Pattern of thinking)
What goes into you: Meals, medics, or anxiety, & sugar	**What you do to refresh your mind:** Yog/pranayam, or wine, & vacation	**How you behave with yourself:** Follow inner voice, or take one more drink	**Thoughts to tickle you:** Solve or Find fault, Arguing who is right, or what is right

- Evolving means self-care at a higher level, including choices in four (4) areas I, II, III, and IV. Most people believe that focusing on a good diet alone will guarantee a happy life. However, as the face is an index to mind, the balanced action in all four areas is an index to total health.

- Yoga practices are designed to remove any imbalance.

- A Japanese researcher has concluded that I + II constitute 30% success and that III + IV are 70%. The latter is the victory of personal values called Jay in Sanskrit. Jay elevates from inside, and you must win.

- Vijay I + II is victory in the external struggle as in a court case. You may win or lose; it depends on the case's merit, presented by the witness and attorneys on both sides.

- Similarly, each person, despite their unique strength and weakness, is capable of paying attention to the inner voice coming from the heart. Honor it like a retired parent living in your home.

- Sundar Pichai, CEO of Google, observed 'Your biggest competition is from within, do not focus on wrong things and get distracted. Success comes from chasing what makes you good as a company.'

- Ajinkya Rahane, India's Captain (Ind vs. Aus 3rd Cricket Test in Sidney), said on day 4 (Jan-11, 2021) 'when set out to bat, India came with a clear plan to fight till the end, and not think about the result.' The match ended in a draw, which was hailed equally to winning.

11. FOOD IS MEDICINE- CHALLENGE YOUR KNOWLEDGE OF DIET

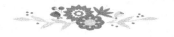

Rules of Yogic Eating	Rules of Yogic Drinking
i) Try not to skip a meal, except on fasting.	i) Avoid carbonated drinks, soda, and ice cream, particularly at mealtime.
ii) Eat when you feel hungry.	ii) Drink only warm water when thirsty
iii) Eat what is nutritious, and eat well and in time. A whole-grain chapati and freshly made vegetable, dal/curry meal cures insomnia.	iii) Drink warm water one hour after or before the meal.
iv) Defeat the urge to emotional eating.	iv) Take buttermilk spiced with *ajwaian,* black pepper, and black salt at lunchtime, and drink hot almond milk with *haldi* at bedtime.
v) Divide the total calories, say 1800 per day, equally among fats, carbs, and proteins (600 each)	v) Alternate to black tea: Try *tulsi-*tea prepared by boiling fresh *tulsi* or herbs in water.
vi) Eat 30 grams of fiber in a day. Every 10 grams added makes you 2-3 years younger in a lifetime.	vi) Read the Nutrition Label before buying a food packet. If unable to work out the arithmetic, **do not buy** that packet
vii) Know by heart the calorie formula 1 g carb, or protein = 4 calories, fat = 9 calories	Be creative. - Top a toast with a slice of fresh fruit in place of peanut butter jelly.
viii) Make 'No Added Sugar' your health mantra.	- A typical recipe for preparing a sugar-free Semolina Halwa dessert dish is attached.
- Avoid substitute sweetener, brown sugar, or honey, and all non-dairy coffee creamers	
- Instead, use Almond milk or evaporated skim milk	
- Cook a dessert made of apples, sweet potato, and	

carrots, or eat pitted dates and bananas at a party. **TIP:** Buy the best quality ingredients.	*Your talent is God's gift to you. What you do with it is your gift back to God* *- **Leo Buscaglia***

Ayurvedic Menu for healthy living

Ayurvedic Halwa- No sugar added (**Serves 4**)

Ingredients

- 2 c water & 2 c whole milk (divided);

- 2 c sweet fruit (thinly sliced dates, raisins, carrots, peeled/shredded apples, ½ c each), 120 gm ghee

- 1 cup (semolina coarse-grained); 1/3 cup walnut pieces, 8- green cardamom- roasted/powdered

Method

- Combine 2 c water, 1 c milk, dates, raisins, carrot, and apples in a 2-quart saucepan.

- Turn to moderate heat. Bring to boil, simmer for 15 min. -Remove from heat and cover with a lid.

- When cooled, mix with a hand blender. This is sweet pulp, with no sugar added.

- Melt the ghee in a 3-quart non-stick saucepan, stir-fry the grains on low heat until fully aromatic.

- Add walnut pieces halfway thru the roasting process.

- Now, turn on the heat under the sweet pulp pan, and bring it to a rolling boil.

- Slowly and steadily pour the hot pulp into the pan of roasted semolina. The grains may stumble at first but quickly stop as the liquid is absorbed.

- Continue stirring. Add milk.

- Sprinkle slivered almonds,

- **Halwa is ready**

Note: For Dudhi halwa, replace Semolina with grated Dudhi.

Ayurvedic Khichdi (Serves 4)

Ingredients

- 1 c yellow Moong dal, 1 c basmati rice

- in pc of fresh ginger, peeled/chopped

- 2 tbsp of dry coconut shreds

- 2 tbsp Fresh cilantro leaves

- 1 Fresh tomato diced; 2- tbsp of ghee

- 2-in piece Cinnamon bark, 5-cloves; 5- cardamom pods, 10- black peppercorns, cumin seeds 1tsp, 3-bay leaves; ½- tsp turmeric powder 1/2-tsp salt, 6 c water; 1 c eggplant cubed, to lower vata, and kapha

Method

- Wash dal and rice 3 times until the water is clear. Soak for 3 hours in warm water for better digestion

- Add ghee, salt, turmeric, and water to the daal, and saute till yellow froth forms. Remove the froth.

- chop ginger, coconut, cilantro, and tomato.

- Set the Instant pot on saute, add ghee, cinnamon, bay leaves, cumin, and peppercorns, and stir till fragrant. Add the chopped items, incl. Eggplant.

- Pressure Cook in 10 minutes - Let it cool down on its own.

- **Khichdi is ready to serve**

TIP: A human being is born with an allotted quota of morsels, breaths, and karmas. Act wisely to extend your physical and mental life spans to fulfill the allotted karmas and re-birth in a better setting.

12. SENIOR FITNESS

Air India failed to recruit physically fit employees from their office staff in Feb. 2019.

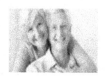

'Age is no more a number'- hints at the role of diet/nutrition, body weight, restorative sleep

Fitness parameter	Fitness Index/ Asana pose	Range of Acceptance	Functional relations in daily life
- Breathing - Posture - Eating - Drugs	- Sit, stand erect - Inhale/exhale 3 sec - carb, fat, protein - Less Rx, more herbs	- P1, P2, P3, P4 pranayamas - 10 to 12 BPM - Zero 'added sugar.' - take supplements	- Reduced risk of falling - Less fatigue, more energy - Sacrifice the 'Junk' diet - Save money
- Strength	- Tadasan pose - Massage each knee - Wide-angle bend - Sit up (arms on chest) - Arm Curl w/5 lb wt	- Raise arms in 3-sec - Extend & Breathe - 5 reps / 30 sec - 5 reps /ea. 60 sec - 11 to 22 reps/ 30 sec	- Whole-body work-out - Walking/lifting easy & safe - Enter/exit the car safely - Body strength - Lifting grandchildren
- Balance	- Talasan - Virasan (chair) - Utkat aasan	- Maintain for 3-6 sec/ 5 X - Maintain 3-6 sec/5X - Walk-in reverse	- Maneuver in crowds - Walk-in narrow lanes - Lift/carry objects
- Endurance Fitness parameter	- March-in-place - Neck & shoulder movement	- 68 to 115 steps in 1-2 min - Repeat 3x....5 min total - 3 reps CW and CCW	- Walking in public parks - Catching a flight at the airport - For safe driving - Minor home care

Fitness parameter	Fitness Index/ Asana pose	Range of Acceptance	Functional relations in daily life
- Flexibility/ dexterity	- Trikonasan- 1,2 - Garudasan - Hands move in a namaste pose	- Maintain the pose for 6 sec - 3 reps in 30-sec - Twist 90 deg, hold 6 sec	- For upper back strength - Reduces pain in fingers - Upper torso endurance
- relaxation	- Savasana pose	- Start with 5 min/day Goal is 15-20 min/day	- To control stress & gain peace of mind
- Emotional stability	- Side bend, twist - forward bend - tree pose - Anulom/vilom	- 3 reps CW and CCW - Same - Hold in the pose for 5 sec - 7 – 21 cycles	- Balance the emotions. Adjust/improve your behavior - Learn the root cause of Ego
- Spiritual evolving	- Choose the path best suited for you	- 10 minutes or more of meditation twice a day at a regular time	- Clean dishes, make the bed, help your spouse in cooking, & seek a higher purpose in life

Lessons from the Covid Pandemic-

i) The risk of a fatal infection is four times higher for normal healthy people 75 and older than for participants under 65 yr

ii) For seniors with chronic health conditions like high BP, obesity, or lung problems, the risk for 75 y/o jumped thirteenfold

iii) 1% of the US population live in long-term care homes, but they represented 43% of all COVID-19 deaths, as the majority already suffered chronic illnesses and had poor immunity.

iv) Yoga-based exercises, as described above, can improve your overall fitness and reduce the risk of COVID infection, no matter your age group. Choose more asanas to suit your current health condition, ex, constipation.

13. THREE GUNAS (DYNAMIC ATTRIBUTES OF NATURE)

as inertia (Tamas), energy (Rajas), and intelligence (Sattva) [YS 4.32]

But you need to know the combo &-how to balance the gunas*.

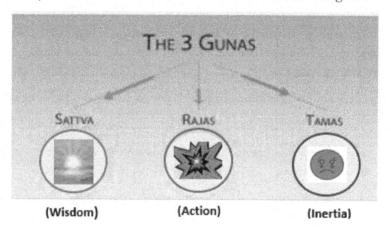

Due to Sattva, we remain conscious and wake up in the morning fresh and ready; it is our potential.

Rajas propel our thoughts, emotions, and feelings to be ready, act, and move; it is the kinetic energy in hand

Because of *Tamas*, we get easily tired or disinterested in creative work and can perform only labor-intensive tasks.

* Firstly, know about yourself which of the three Gunas occupies your mind the bulk of the time? For example

-   If reason succumbs to the pull of greed and restlessness, your feverish act is guided by *Rajas*.

-   If delusion prevails, *Tamas* predominates, and you're misled to imbibe wrong knowledge.

- When *sattva* increases, righteousness (Self-discipline, wisdom, & positivity......) manifests in all actions.

- *sattva* is dominant in a scholar; rajas is dominant in a warrior and takes a back seat in a businessman. In routine laborers, tamas predominate, and sattva plays a lesser role.

• Understanding the three Gunas (tamas, rajas, and sattva), and their variation helps in setting a higher objective in life, beyond trifles such as passing a school examination, securing a job, and building up a bank balance, raising a family, acquiring a house, and stuffing it.

• It is commonly observed that their financial success may not relieve their boredom and dissatisfaction in life for the' successful' industrialists and company executives.

• Three types of people are usually present in the auditorium of the world:

  - *Tamasik* guy sleeps through the show and feeling lazy to watch

  - *Rajasik* person is impatient to get out and work on a business project ahead of others,

  - *Sattvik* is mindful of enjoying the show, having made a choice and paid the price

• The difference between a yogi, an ordinary person, or a rich industrialist is that the yogi judges/makes an effort to know his gunas and upgrade the thoughts before it affects him- an ordinary householder feels good by judging others forgets his nature.

• So, the goal of righteous living is: to correct the guna imbalance.

• If upset, reduce *Tamas*. Stay away from *tamasik* foods, meat dishes, leftovers, and processed or canned stuff. Also, add Rajas- Engage in yoga. Do *Tadasan*, clasp your hands as you lift, followed by five rounds of Sun salutation, which improves breathing, and good mood.

• Balancing *Rajas*? Slow down, Do *Nadi shodhan*, and *Shitali* (cooling breath pranayama). Sit down to eat and chew thoroughly every morsel, stay away from fried foods, and eat leafier and anti-oxidant-rich veggies.

- Cultivating *Sattva*: Eat more fresh foods (plant-based organic diet). Sleep 7-8 hours and wake up at decent times to practice devotion/meditation and spend more time in nature.

14. SEVEN ENERGY CENTERS: CHAKRAS- 101

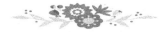

Chakras are gates in the human body; #7 awakens Kundalini's power [1,2,3,4]

Chakra*	Location	Purpose	Asana pose	Affirm
7. Crown (Violet)	Top of head	Kundalini shakti	Meditation	I am
6. Third eye	eye brows	Intuition, Wisdom	Adhomukh	I see
5. Throat	lower mind	Communication	Vipritkarni	I speak
4. Heart	Chest centre	Love, compassion	Sethubandh	I love
3. Solar plexus	Upper belly	Self- esteem	Boat	I can
2. Sacral	Lower belly	Sexuality, creativity	Frog	I feel
1. Root (Red)	Base of spine	Survival, family	Balasan	I wish

1. Muladhar,   2. Swadhistan,   3. Manipur,   4. Anahat,

5. Visudh,   6. Ajya,   7. Sahasrar

*Each Chakra has a color link with the seven colors of the rainbow. VIBGYOR

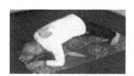
Adho mukh

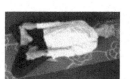
Supt-padmasan

Viprit karni

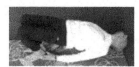
sethu bandhasan

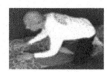
Frog pose

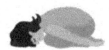
Balasan

(1).   First, learn the chakra where you presently are, suiting to your dosha/temperament.

(2).   Ex: When attached to worldliness, the mind dwells in the lower chakras 1, 2, or 3.

(3). Chakra 4 is the beginning of spiritual awakening. For further progress, do Purity practice.

(4). At chakra 5 (freedom from ignorance/delusion), at 6(direct vision of God), and 7(*samadhi*)

15. PURITY PRACTICE

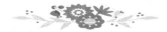

The Sanskrit word is Shauch (# 1 in the list of 5 Niyamas /observances)

PURITY IN THE BODY REALM

Daily Practice

Bowel movement

- Drink 2 cups of warm water in the morning and take a tsp of Triphala powder at bedtime.

Cleaning and oiling the mouth - Gargle with warm salt water

- Use herbal toothpaste

- Rub sesame oil on gums, and weekly gargle in sesame oil

Cleaning and oiling the nose

- Sniff ½ c warm saltwater in the nostrils, or use Jal neti pot

- Dip your pinkie finger in the oil and gently massage inside of the nostrils.

Cold shower

End the shower with a 30-sec cold- water rinse.

Massage the whole Body

Towel gently after the shower, and apply sesame oil to the whole body.

Weekly Practice

Oiling the eyes

Melt a small amount of ghee in a heated spoon. Let 2 drops of cooled ghee fall in each eye.

Oiling the anus

Dip a finger in ½ tsp sesame oil. Then insert the finger to rub 1 inch inside the anus.

Monthly Practice

Oiling the ears

- squeeze 3 drops of sesame oil in one ear, keeping head tilted for 3 minutes; repeat with the other ear. Cleaning the colon

- Practice if constipated, but not more than twice a week

- Take ½ to 1 tsp castor oil two hours before going to bed. Follow with ½ c warm water.

Annually

Shankh prakshalan kriya to clean the alimentary canal.

PURITY AT MIND REALM

Daily on-the-go Practice

- **Love/discover yourself**, perform all actions in the day mindfully- the 3Rs principle

- **Watch your reactions.** Life is 10% what happens to you; 90% is how you make it by the act/react process. Mental cleansing is a sattvic act.

- **It helps in 4 ways:**

    i) You make good habits. Ex. React consciously, not foolishly

    ii) Optimize a mix of three gunas

    iii) You'll no more entertain a tamasik act, to downgrade your spiritual progress, cause hurt on purpose

    iv) You're meditating more often.

Cupping: Stroke the 6 body joints, 30 sec each body joint daily.

Acupressure: Make it a daily routine in the shower to give treatment to areas that hurt.

TIP: In defense of purity at all three realms in the human body, take the example of the Uranium. The ore contains 1% uranium, but it must be processed to 99.9% purity to use as nuclear fuel.

16. ACCESSORIES/SUPPORTS

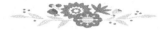

If a pose may cause pain in the joint, try a modification or use a support.

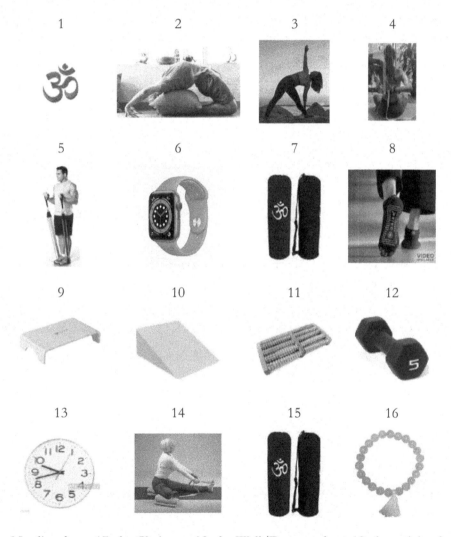

Not listed: no. 17, the Chair, no. 18, the Wall/Door, and no. 19, the weighted blanket for grounding effect

1. AUM	2, 3. Bolster, Foam block	4. Strap	5. Resistance Band	6. Smart watch	7. Tote bag	8. Skid-free shoes
9. Step stool	10. Foam wedge	11. Foot Massager	12. 5-lb weight	13. Wall clock,	14. Strap & Blanket 15. Yoga mat	16. Rosary/ Japa mala

TIP: Listen, and honor your innate uniqueness. Soon you will discover the right stretch as well as the support. For Chair yoga, consciously choose the chair height and cushion, treating the chair as an extension of your legs.

Legend: Topic 16. Con.t from

1. AUM - the symbol kept at eye level increases awareness of the Divine presence in you.

2. FOAM BLOCK

3. Bolster increases your capacity to stretch your body in difficult asanas.

4. STRAP- increases the reach in challenging poses, ex. Paschimottanasan

5. RESISTANCE BAND- 30 LB capacity is handy for conditioning the legs.

6. SMARTWATCH- helps monitor the progress and adjust the stretch to a safe level.

7. TOTE BAG- a better way to carry the devices around from home to the yoga studio.

8. SKID-FREE SOCKS/ SHOES- safe legs are stretching as in warrior pose or Forward Bend pose.

9. STEP STOOL- 8 in rising for practicing going up or down the stairs. Also, use Foot Roller 11.

10. FOAM WEDGE- Sitting on the floor with a wedge underneath to keep hips and knees at the level

11. MASSAGER- 10- min practice massages the soles & palms at all acupressure points

12. 5-LB WEIGHT- Strength training of arms, even when sitting in a chair

13. WALL CLOCK to sync your breathing with mantra, moves, and clicking of seconds

14. BLANKET- For support of knees or standing on all fours. Ex. Dog-Cat pose.

15. YOGA MAT- Buy a nice, slip-free, thin mat of natural fiber and easy to carry on the shoulder

16. ROSARY- Japa Mala- use it to count time and breaths in meditation practice.

TIP: An average healthy person takes ~ 700 million breaths in the life span of 75 years.

Proper posture, deep breathing & silence in one hour of yoga can add up to 5 more years.

17. PATANJALI'S YOG-DARSHAN 2000-YEAR-OLD BOOK

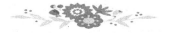

The proven way to Know God thru yoga

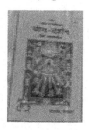

8 Steps to enlightenment [YS II.29]

8. SAMADHI- Spiritual union

7. DHYANA- Meditation

6. DHARANA- Concentration

5. PRATYAHAR- Sense withdrawal by will

4. PRANAYAMA- Measured Breathing

3. ASANA- Sit upright, with tall spine
2. NIYAMA-5 rules to make good habits
1. YAMA- 5 vows to cleanse out bad habits

5 Yama (restraints): non-injury, truth, non-covetousness, chastity in thought/deed, and not expecting material gift (ready for step 2)
5 Niyama (observances): purity, contentment, austerity, and Self-study for personal growth, and trust in God (ready for step 3)

(195) aphorisms divided in four chapters

I. Samadhi Pada.... Aims   (51)

II. Sadhana Pada.. Practices   (55)

III. Vibhuti Pada.... Powers   (55)

IV. Kaivalya Pada.... Liberation (34)

Note: 1 aphorism from each chapter

YS I.24 *Purush-Vishesh Isvarah*
Where Consciousness is, God is.

YS II.46 *Sthir sukhamasanam*
Posture should be steady and comfortable.

YS III.26 *Bhuvan jnanam suryesanyamat*
Gain cosmic knowledge by focusing on the Sun

YS IV.30 *Tatah kleshakarma nivritti*
As grace descends, klesha and karma are washed off

- yamas are moral ethics: ahimsa, satya, asteya, brahmcharya, aparigrah – similar to removing weeds

- niyamas are good habits: shauch, santosh, tap, swadhyay, ishvar pranidhana- similar to sowing new seeds

- Yamas Niyamas are the ten rules of successful living, but not enough to know God or the way to the higher life.

Hence, sage Patanjali added six more steps: #3 to steady the body (asana), #4 to quiet the mind (pranayama), #5, #6 for Concentration, contemplation (pratyahara, dharna), #7 for meditation (dhyana), and #8 for self-absorption(samadhi).

The group of eight steps is popularly known as Ashtang Yoga or Raj yoga.

Patanjali's Yog Darshan, the book of eight limbs, continues to appeal even today.

From practical considerations and time constraints, you may simultaneously practice 3Rs, and steps 3 and 4. This is good for sense control- Salient components are Purity practice (Nauli), Asana postures (sarvangasan, Viprit Karni), Pranayama (Nadi shodhan), and meditation (dhyan).

The shortcut is relevant in modern times too. It assists in making day-to-day decisions, such as choosing an academic career, choosing a teacher, selecting a spouse, setting up a family, or shedding 10 lb to look good at an upcoming family event, finally leaving more time for spiritual growth.

How to be Spiritual is everyone's dilemma. As you control the thought waves and emotions, do asanas, and meditate daily, you will get correct answers to your query.

There is a sutra [YS 4.4] Nirman chittany asmitamatrat. All man-created ripples in the consciousness proceed from fake ego. There is another beautiful sutra YS I.27 'The word which expresses God is OM,' and I.28 'This word must be repeated with meditation/affirmation upon its meaning'. Such chanting changes the climate of your mind from negative to positive. It is practical! Ex: Refer to [YS I.7] Pratyakshanumanagama pramanani on three proofs of right knowledge

i)   Direct perception(pratyaksh): right knowledge begins with seeing and believing

ii) Inference(anuman): intellect also needs inferential reasoning, like smoke infers fire

iii) Scriptural testimony (Aagam): expert advice offered by a guru is also important. It happened to me!

While buying our starter home in New Jersey in 1985, my wife and I took three sensible steps before signing the formal contract (then, we had not known about sage Patanjali)

i)   looked into newspaper ads and visited three homes (pratyaksh)

ii) consulted friends, local school, and police station to make an inference (anuman)

iii) obtained a written report from a licensed inspector, qualified home appraiser (agam)

18. POPULAR YOGA PATHS & MODES OF POSTURES

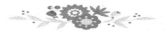

Ref. 1, p.136 lists over 500 Asana postures. The following short list is presented for seniors

No	7 Popular Yoga paths	11 Posture modes	(31) Popular Asanas/postures
01	Raj yoga- 8 limb tradition of sage Patanjali	1.Grounding	BEGIN Pray/Sit, Tadasan, Yastikasan (3)
02	Karma yoga- path of Action for active mind	2. Warming	Dog/Cat pose, Chakrasan Variations (2)
		3. Balancing	Ekpadasan, Talasan (2)
03	Bhakti yoga- path of Devotion for choice god	4. Strengthening	Adhomukh, Svan pose, Warrior 1, 2 (4)
		5. Backward bending	Bhujangasan, Bridge, Bow, Locust, Fish (5)
04	Hath yoga -from body and breath to Raj yoga	6. Forward bending	Balasan, Manduk, Paschim otan(3)
		7. Inverting	Vipritkarni, Halaasan (2)
05	Iyengar yoga – emphasize detail, precision and props	8. Twisting	Konasan, Matsyendra, Parsvkonasan (3)
06	Kundalini- Specialized method of self-realization	9. Hip opening	Butterfly, Lunge, Gomukhasan, Pigeon (4)
		10. All of above	Surya Namaskar, Sarvangasan (2)
07	Vinyas- breathing & music	11. Relax	Savasan (Corpse pose) (1) END

Note 1: The eBook suggests selected Asanas with conscious breathing.
Note 2: Also, smiling/ affirming helps gain efficiency in-home or at work.

At the end of an Asana, observe moments of silence and sensation as an aid to consciousness.

TIP: Better call these- yoga pills and meditation pills. Learn which yoga and when? You must decide which poses are apt for you. Remember, each pose is not good for you.

19.1 BUILD DAILY HOME PRACTICE (20 MIN/DAY)

5-steps to a yogic lifestyle for being socially/physically active

S. No.	Sequence
1.	BEGIN AUM chant 3X
2.	Basic Pranayamas P1...P4
3.	Sun salutation in chair 5X
4.	Meditation
5.	Prayer sit-in pose END

19.2 CURE FOR
ANXIETY/HYPERTENSION/HIGH BP

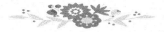

Determine the root cause of the high BP-study the relation between Nature and You

- Kapha dosha is related to increased viscosity of the blood

- Pitta dosha is responsible for increased force/velocity of blood

- Vata dosha for seniors > 65 y/o causes thickening of blood vessels

The following yogic remedies will heal and gradually reduce the dosage of prescribed Rx medicines.

- **shitali pranayama** (make a tube of your tongue, and inhale deeply into the abdomen), hold briefly, and exhale slowly thru the nose. Repeat 8X.

- Choose the poses that put the spine horizontal and the heart is below the spine, similar to animals.

   Surya namaskar in a chair, child pose, dog/cat pose, one-legged stretch (janu shirasan), gentle hip openers (frog pose/baddha konasan), sit in nishpandbhav, and end in meditation and prayer.

   TIP: Add mulbandh root lock in exhale, when possible.

- Be gentle, slow, and rhythmic. Caution: Avoid headstands, weight lifting, or vigorous exercise that causes extreme discomfort and breathlessness. Be smart; use supports, foam blocks, or chairs.

* TIPS: While yoga is for everyone, every Asana/Pranayama is not for everyone.

19.3 BUILD HOME PRACTICE (1-HR) FOR TOTAL HEALTH

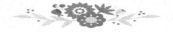

No two persons are alike, yet everyone has similar aspirations-

Fit body, Rhythmic breathing, Cool mind, Kind heart & Awakened spirit

(Pusth sharir, Sangitmay svas, Ekagra mann, Unnat bhav, Chetan shakti)

- BEGIN Aum chant 3X .... 5 minutes
- Warm-up Breathing (P1, P2, P3, P4) .... 4 minutes
- Warm-up Surya namaskar in chair-12 poses .... 6 minutes
- Therapeutic Asanas for Strength, Endurance, Balance*...... 20 minutes
- Therapeutic Pranayama.. 15 minutes
    - Brahm kriya, Anulom/Vilom
    - Bhramari, and Kapaalbhati
    - Ear, eye, neck, hands, feet care. OK, to use a strap to stretch the hands/feet
- Acupressure and/or cup therapy
- Meditation .... 5 - 10 minutes
- Yogic Prayer .... END

* (Vajrasan, Balasan, Spinal twist, Dog/Cat, Ardh Chandrasan, yog mudra, Sethubandhasan, Sarvangasan, Pavanmuktasan, Hanumanasan - total 10 poses)

TIP: If the body is strong & mind is calm, you are prompted to speak the truth. [Vigyanmay kosha]

19.4 BUILD HOME PRACTICE FOR PROSTATE HEALTH

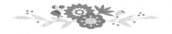

1. **Common symptoms**

    -   70% of men over 60 experience enlarged benign prostate gland, called BPH

    -   (gland's weight gain 20 g-100 g)

    -   The problem may begin at age 50, causing frequent urination, especially at night

    -   Pain while emptying the bladder

    Natural care/cures-

    -   If PSA rises, check every six months for cancer specificity and kidney damage.

    -   Eat drink responsibly/stay warm

    -   Acupressure treatment on the wrist area

    -   Treat bedtime meditation to a sleeping pill

    -   Visit restroom often in-home or office.

2. **Yoga is exercise at a subtle level**

    Every man should do yoga

    -   Avoid high impact jogging or cycling

    -   Recommend brisk walking outdoors

    -   Else walk on the treadmill, but no jogging

    -   Do Ashwini mudra in sitting (pulling or sucking the anus inward in a series of tense-release movements). Repeat 10X.

    -   Do 10-min yoga each time you wake up as gratitude to your body at night.

Side benefits: better sleep, better digestion, instant boost of the mood

How to sit? Sit in Padmasana or Sukh Asan pose on the floor; sit erect and avoid cross-legged if in a chair.

3. **Poses in sitting**

   ### 3.1 Balasan (child pose)

   - Sit in Vajrasan (hero) pose

   - Exhale, do Ashwini mudra, and kneel forward

   - Exhale once more, continue to kneel, and stretch your arms on the floor in front, for 10-20 seconds

   3.2 Nishpand bhav - is an effective, easy pose. Sit against the wall, spreading your legs wide.

   Try one leg at a time, the other leg folded. Soon, you can spread both legs, stay in pose 5 min followed by Badh konasan for 2-3 minutes

   3.3 Shalabhasan- Very effective, combines strength, balance, and endurance. Hold 1 min.

   OK, to use bolster below thighs.

4. **Legs up the wall**

   - Sit in a comfortable pose near the wall. Lie down, and simultaneously legs move up on the wall

   - Keep a bolster under the butts. This is a relaxing master pose if you can breathe deep for 2 minutes without holding.

5. **Pose in lying down on the belly**

   ### 5.1 Dhanurasan (bow pose)

   - Belly hugging the floor, inhale, bend and try catching legs in the shape of a bow

   - feel energetic, ready to take aim

   - Exhale and relax

6. **Poses in standing**

   6.1 Surya namaskar (11 poses in chair)

   - add root lock in exhale

   6.2 Agnisar kriya

   - Bend at knee/hip, thighs, and torso 90o

   - Exhale in steps, apply Root lock, churning stomach, total 10 cycles

   6.3 Oil massage

   - Gently massage sesame oil to the prostate area. First in a circular motion, then stroke from the anus to the base of the penis. Do not press hard.

7. **Diet and Conclusions**

   - Eat foods rich in zinc, ex—pumpkin seeds and tomatoes every day (you lose 15 mg of zinc each urination).

     Reduce alcohol intake, red meat, and eggs.

   - Change diet to vegan.

   - Eat whole wheat than rice at dinner.

   - Avoid dairy; rather, Drink almond milk.

   - Drink less fluid after 6 pm. Drink slowly.

   - Drink mostly warm water when thirsty.

   - Even women should learn; they can teach an uncle, brother, or friend. Be kind to others.

   - Prefer Yoga to any exercise.

Progress may be slow, but it is certain.

19.5 HOME CARE FOR SPINE HEALTH-TWIST & BEND

Observe Sensations of well-being

1. Tadasan............................... Namaste & Twist Variant

2. Sarvangasan.......................... Lie down and raise on shoulders

3. Utkatasan............................ Stand & Twist in Chair pose

4. Vakrasan............................. Sitting on the floor & twist

5. Lotus pose w/Twist................ Sitting on the floor & twist

6. Supta-vakrasan..................... Lying pose, in a twist

7. Parsva Balasan...................... Child pose in Vajrasan &Twist

8. Janu Savasan........................ Revolved head/knee pose

9. Supta Garudasan.................. Lying pose, Twist hands & feet

1	2	3

4	5	6

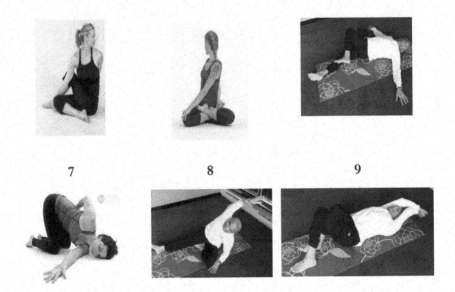

7   8   9

19.6 SELECTED ASANAS FOR YOUNG ADULTS/STUDENTS

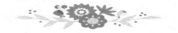

If State can mandate the **COVID** vaccine for school students, why not introduce yoga in schools?

The biggest gain of yoga is emotional well-being and inclusive awareness

- **kapalrandhra dhouti** for body awareness: **Sukhasan & Savasan** for relaxation

- **Nishpandbhava** for sensitivity, **Ekpadasan** for steadiness, **Parvatasan** for flexibility

- **Stithprarathnasan/Talasan** for co-ordination, **Virasan** to be ready for action

- **Vajrasan** sit straight up often, **Ardhapadmasan** sits for concentration

- **Yogmudra** for humility, **Utkatasan** for skill in the execution of the assigned task

- **Pranayama** P1, P2, P3, and P4 for healthy breathing and to build immunity

- **Anulom/Vilom** for better breathing to resolve conflicts in small groups

- **Silence/simple** meditation to improve focus in studies and avoid depression

- **Picnic & stories** for training in healthy relationship, aka inclusiveness

20. UPASANA – PRAYER

Every positive thought is a prayer. A prayer is answered when done with devotion, like children

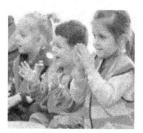 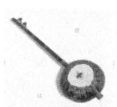

| Children praying | *Ektara* playing |

- **BEGIN**: YOG class begins with 3 Aum chants in a sitting *namaste* pose

  Then the hands, eyes, and tongue are positioned not to distract 3-5 sec deep inhale lets life-force flow to every limb of the body & Exhale in 6-10 sec, to get all stale air out of the lungs: a 2-in-1 kriya

- **END**: The following Vedic prayer ends the class.

May we move in harmony and speak in unison	**Samgacchadhvam, samvadadhvam**
May our minds are in equanimity as in the beginning	**sam vo manāmsi jānatām, devā bhāgam yathā pūrve**
May divinity manifest in all our endeavors.	**sañjānānā upāsate**

- Smiling, clapping (acupressure treatment is a side benefit), & counting with Chanting 'Aum 1, 2, 3, 4 for hearing signals in the heart (inner voice).

- Chant Gayatri mantra in 16-sec, 8-sec, or 4-sec, as needed.

- Sit steady, and observe the *kirtan* stance of body/mind in harmony

- Make mental humming your background *Ektara* music during the day.

21. MANTRA, PRAYER & MEANING

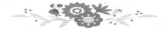

Just as the human body needs food, the soul/spirit needs prayer

- No matter what material wealth you possess, peace of mind can be attained only in prayer. You are blessed with strength and wisdom when you think of Aum with genuine feeling.

- NASA's modern science has discovered that AUM prayer is ongoing in the hottest core of the sun. The trees, plants, birds, and butterflies also flutter in Aum.

Make AUM your new prayer to regulate blood pressure, heartbeat, sleep, study, and bowel habits.

AUM is the shortest holy mantra, but there are other popular Mantras -

1. *AUM*........................... 1 sec   **4.** *So Hum*................. 1 - 2 sec

2. *Aum Namo Shivaya*.........…..... 3 sec   **3.** *Gayatri Mantra*…….….…..8 sec

5. *Aum Bhur Bhuva Svaha*......2 - 4 sec   **6.** *Hanuman chalisa*……......…5 min

- Correct pronouncing and understanding the subtle meaning enhances the mantra effect. Use the following examples of non-stop chants-

    - going upstairs (*AUM, AUM, AUM*......)

    - raising the arms in 2-sec warm-up pose (*AUM 1, AUM 2*),

    - twisting the torso 90 deg in vakrasan in 3 sec (*Aum Tat Sat*)

    - doing sun salutation (*Full Gayatri mantra*)

    - taking a shave (Gayatri Mantra multiple times), -taking a shower (*Hanuman Chalisa*)

Once or twice a day, laugh vigorously for 30 sec/2 Gayatri chants or muktahaas , or lion pose.

TIP: If you do not get a razor cut on the face or feel safer walking, take it as a mantra effect.

Make the daily goal: 1008 Gayatri chants, which is a miracle! I DO IT; YOU CAN DO IT.

22. CONCLUSION: PART TWO

Yoga is real Fun in Senior years

In Nature's fascinating design- a human being is fully equipped to live healthy for up to 100 years. But how?

- Do yoga to keep the body moving, mind to be calm, and meditate in silence.

- Also, you'll do every little Act in a manner that brings you closer to the inner Spirit.

  Take 1 small step, and the supreme God takes 9. Ex. Draupadi summoned Krishna in Mahabharata

- Join a YOG group – upgrade each act, thought, or feeling to a higher level and keep going forward. [for the list of divine & demoniacal properties]

- Take care of the health issues affecting seniors by doing proper Asanas

i) Psychiatric disorders- causing dementia, and depression…......…...........

ii) Respiratory issues- breathing difficulty, COPD…...……...…..............

iii) Mental turmoil - stress, loneliness, heart disease, cancer, diabetes…...

iv) Oral hygiene- bathing, purity practice, & the routine diagnostic tests…...

v) Osteoporosis - loss of bone density, fractures, and joint disorder…...…....….........….

vi) Circulatory system/metabolism, and constipation….…….................

vii) Vision and hearing loss …...…..........

viii) Memory loss …..…........

- A short skirt may be enough to cover the essentials, but the 9-yard saree is needed to decorate the body gracefully.

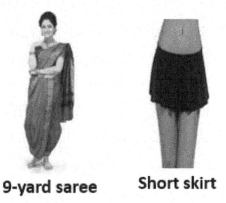

9-yard saree   **Short skirt**

- Similarly, decorate the mind and heart with good thoughts, mantras, or humming poetry music playing in the background.

REFRESH THE BASICS

- All human beings are born unique, yet their basic aims are to eat, drink and make merry.

  To most people, health means making money & seeing the doctor when ill, getting cured, and re-start.

- A few ~ 4% realize the need to do yoga by WhatsApp, visit studios, and read free magazines.

  Half of this 1 – 2 % may realize Total health is different - how to prevent from falling ill or recover faster.

- There are 7 yogic paths, 11 yoga-posture types, and 31 yog asasanas listed in the eBook

- Consult a licensed teacher and avoid random workouts in a gym for the right choice!

  Smart means using support/accessories if needed to make the asanas joyful and without fatigue.

  Conscious means making rhythmic breathing and chanting an integral part of body movement.

- Surya namaskar 5 – 12 rounds on the chair are strongly recommended every morning.

- You can combine the bending, twisting, stretching, backward and forward poses- in either standing, sitting, or lying down postures. Be innovative and creative. Listen to your body/mind

- Follow the 3Rs for consciousness/mindfulness/swabhiman/+ve ego building.

- Your health improves as the urge for wrong food and wrong emotions no more boss over your mind. Other people would not dictate your well-being. Finally, You're in control of yourself.

TIP: Redeem your rights to gain the right knowledge (praman) and avoid wrong knowledge(vipryay).

Then, a yog-trained student studies harder, a retiree is no more a couch potato, a manager finds more time to enjoy with the family, and a prisoner is reformed to be law-abiding.

- Yogic concepts are like Mission Statement in an organization or the initial wedding wows; not many, however, care to review the document later.

Ordinary Lifestyle – Be safe/selfish, & Survive	Yogic Lifestyle – Be loving/selfless, & Thrive
Eat, drink & die	Evolve, transform, & pass
Diet should be organic and tasty, if tamasic, So what?	Diet must be sattvic, nutritious, and freshly cooked
Fearful in life and death: the suffering of mental, cardiovascular, obesity, diabetes	Fit body, calm mind, and manage the allotted time fear-free

- A yogi's creativity is expressed in performing a Yogasana, stretching more than one body part at a time. Sarvangasan, suryanamaskar, and pranayama are boons to humanity, a panacea for the most common human ailments.

- On the contrary, a raw 'unyogic' mind fails to caution the mouth to stay away from 'junk' food.

- Ex. The sweet Tic-Tac mints may provide a temporary or illusory feeling of being okay, which doesn't last or nourish. Rather it depletes energy and wastes the hard-earned money too.

- After taking a shower, I do 'cupping therapy for the six body joints- 1/2 minute for each joint, plus at the naval and medulla behind the head.

- Simultaneously, singing Gayatri Mantra makes cupping more effective.

- Also, do the cupping on any body part needing instant relief, incl. palming the eyes

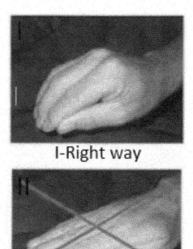

I-Right way

PART THREE:

HOW TO YOGA?

1. MAKE YOG A SUBTLE, HIGHER STYLE OF HEALING

In the USA: 83 million COVID-19 cases and over 1 million deaths and rising. The federal gov't spent $3.4 trillion on public health care in 2021, more than double in 2019

- More cases of mental health, resulting in more deaths and more suicides. Life expectancy fell 1.5 years in 2020, the lowest since 2003. Despite the uncertainty and chaos, yoga stood out as a saviour.

1. Make protocols a new lifestyle now and ever after

   - Be creative, plan your daily tasks lovingly, and skilfully

   - Ex.1 Travel if you must; otherwise, stay well at home to develop new skills

   - Ex.2 WhatsApp messages: delete what hurt, but don't get mad or sad

2. Know what is preventable, and act early to 'nip the evil in the bud.'

   - Why delay doctor visits, annual shots, or yoga practice

3. Going Digital is the futuristic need of humanity

   - Wellness and wireless are inter-linked for mass vaccination in a limited time.

4. Invoke DI: Divine Intervention compliments individual effort

   - Covid-19 proved how science & spirituality speeds healing.

   - Treat life as a lease contract with God

2. CELEBRATING YOG

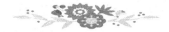

- An Evening of Live Show

- YOG Dance (10 min)

- Demo YOG Poses (25 min)

- Chair YOG (25 min)

- Putting YOG to Remedial work- wall posters

- Pizza party

TIP: Every survivor of war, illness, or calamity has a story laced with divine intervention

Therefore, make yoga your choice of worship and feel instantly better.

Ex: When you practice non-violence (ahimsa), Yama (restraint) # 1 only for a week, as part of a planned sabbatical, you'll observe the following improvements in your lifestyle

Body (physical) non-violence - **not eat** late at night, avoid stale food, meat dishes, alcohol, etc

Mind (mental) non-violence - **not feel bad** when something someone said you didn't like, **overcome** thoughts that stem from negative emotions/samskaras, **and avoid** violent acts

Spiritual non-violence - **stop hate;** instead, pray for love for yourself and all living beings; **care for nutrition** to body, mind, and spirit too

3. INDIVIDUAL VS. COLLECTIVE KARMA

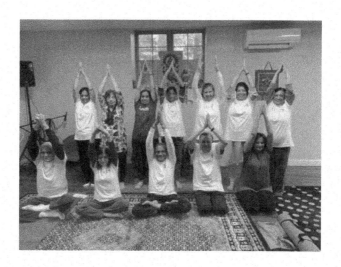

Why the collective celebration?

YOG at an individual level heals a person, but in a group heals the people. The curve moves from -ve on the left to +ve on the right.

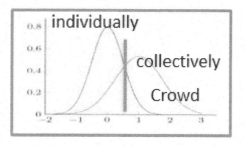

Individually each one is different, not better or worse. Accept this fact for more mutual tolerance and better healthcare too.

Emphasis shifts from my individual karma to <u>our</u> collective karma.

Ex.1: The safety of women and children in the community must involve the town to share responsibility.

Ex.2: At a traffic signal, it is your civic duty to honor the lights turning green to orange to red, regardless of whether the traffic cop is there. Surely, accidents are reduced, and the society gains.

4. YOG IS DANCE

WELCOME………….. Ravi Rustagi Choreographer…….Jayu Parikh

What are Sync and Balance?

'Sync' is an abbreviation of synchronicity, when body, mind, and heart work in unison.

More so in YOG Dance, when the physical moves and gestures of individual members (there were 25), the music and the lights played in complete harmony. Example of a synced mouse to the computer.

mouse

Kudos to Jayu Parikh, the esteemed choreographer.

In YOG practice, sync connotes harmony between the body's movement, the rhythm of breathing, and Japa chant in the heart. Then the benefits from the same pose add up.

Sync is also associated with regularity, similar to the natural phenomena, rising or setting of the sun, tidings of the ocean waves, and weather changes. Studies of the habits of centenarians suggested that people who live long and in good health have had a regular lifestyle since their adulthood. They also spend time in the community, consistently eat quality meals, meditate and go to bed regularly, in sync with circadian rhythms.

'Balance' means your left foot and right foot exert equal 50 – 50 pressures while standing in the Tadasana pose. You twist equally well to your left as well as right.

With regular care in the mid-age, your body parts retain balance and flexibility, and many preventable sicknesses associated with old age can be avoided. Then you age gracefully.

4. YOG IS DANCE

TIP: To enjoy the golden years, a yogic lifestyle must be acquired before retiring.

5. YOG IS FUN

SEQUENCE OF DEMO ASANAS (Mix of Chair & Floor Poses)

Practice 1 hour/day for 21 days, then you get bonded to Yog, and get up to 700% ROI

YOG IS **CONSCIOUS FUN** - FOR TOTAL HEALTH

YOG IS **OUR BUSINESS** - TO BE HEALTHY & WEALTHY

YOG IS **ALL DAY WORK** - DYNAMIC & TRANSFORMING

YOG IS **EFFORT & KNOWLEDGE** BASE IMPROVING

YOG IS **FULL 5-COURSE MENU** FOR NOURISHING THE

BODY, MIND, INTELLECT, HEART & SOUL SPIRIT

TIP- Earn & redeem rewards toward a richer life

America is rich and a spend-thrift nation- spending 95% of Its healthcare budget on treating illnesses and less than 5% on staying well and preventing illness.

Yoga shows the way. Celebrating June 21 as International Yoga Day

Is certainly not enough.

TIP-India and USA can steer the world in the right direction

Be creative & enjoy the game.......

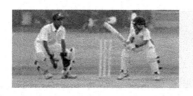

- Sit upright in a sturdy chair, or march in place

- keep fingers in vayu or gyan mudra

- Inhale/exhale normally in nose

- Exercise the neck with eyes wide open

- When a wicket falls, or a boundary is scored, clap n acupressure till the next player comes

- In advt. time, take a break, move hands, fingers, & legs in your favorite warm-up pose

- when thoughts distract, return to the game

- The game is not over till the last ball is played. **A great lesson in witnessing and patience!**

6. LIST OF 28 CONTRIBUTORS

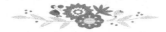

No.	Name	No.	Name
1	Sheetal Patel	15	Rajal Kusumgar
2	Manda Shah	16	Kokila Jani
3	Harsh Jerath	17	Kirit Kothari
4	Surekha Khedekar	18	Minesh Kusumgar
5	Tarun Mehta	19	Arun Mama Yagnik
6	Dashrath Jani	20	Surendra Jain
7	Avinash Jerath	21	Jatin Gajarawala
8	Kalpana Gajarawala	22	Daksha Patel
9	Vimal Narang	23	Anita Sethi
10	Divya Patel	24	Jagdish Shah
11	Dileep Khedekar	25	Raksha Gajarawala
12	Shilpa Mehta	26	Jayu Parikh
13	Nilaxi Bhatt	27	Dilip Parikh
14	Swati Kothari	28	Rayna Rustagi

7. DEMO POSTURES

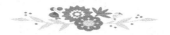

Chair Pose

Forward Bend

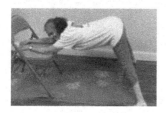

Benefits

- Instant relief in backache

- Keeps back slouch-free

- Strengthens whole body

- Improves Balance

- Opens groin, hamstrings

Eagle pose

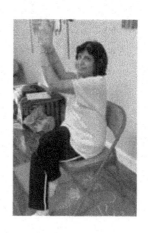

Benefits

- Relieves pain in hands/feet

- Spine is strengthened

Pigeon pose

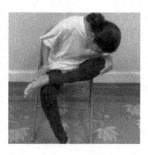

Let the torso move down, and lift the left knee as far as convenient.

Benefits

- Cures abdominal pain

- Strengthens legs / spine

Spinal twist

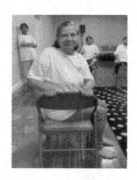

Benefits

- Tones the breathing

- Strengthens spine

- shoulders aligned

Trikonasan (Extended side angle)

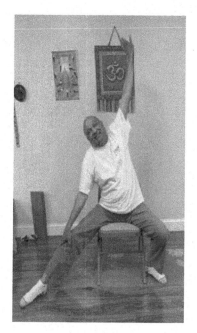
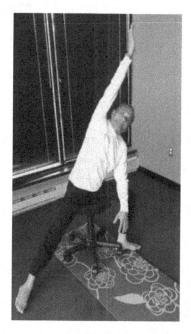

Early variation   Final pose

Dog-cat

chair pose

Dog pose   Cat pose

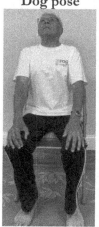
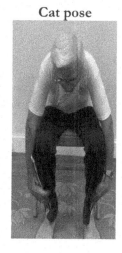

Floor pose

Dog pose

Cat pose

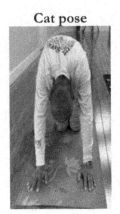

Dog pose: Begin in a tabletop position. Inhale to arch your back concave, and drop the belly downward. Maintain spine length throughout. Gaze upward on 3rd eye.

Cat pose: Exhale and relax your back, make it a convex shape, and gaze below

Talasan pose

Chair pose

Floor pose

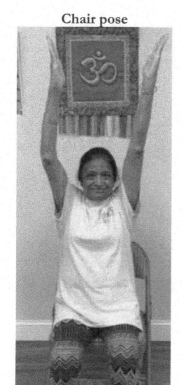
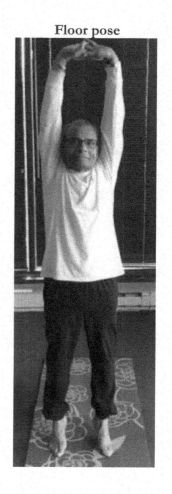

Same as Tadasan pose,

Benefits

- Upper body stretches

- Tones spine

- Improves Balance

- May raise one hand at a time

Pigeon pose

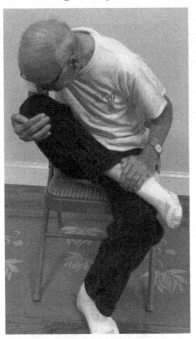

Meditation in chair

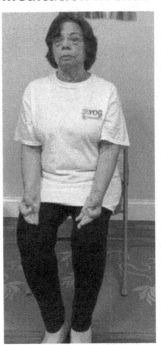

Sit in a chair. Bend your right knee, and grasp the ankle to rest on the left thigh. Draw your chin toward your chest without bending the neck. Hold for 3-6 breaths. Repeat the other side.

- Strengthens legs which sit the whole day

- It Opens the chest & shoulders

Warrior, I pose

- Begin in Tadasan pose, with your hands, on your hips

- Walk your legs apart 3 ft

- Right foot to the front, and Left foot ~ 45^0

- Bend the right leg as you inhale, pressing all 4 corners of both feet into the mat

- Raise hands to elongate the torso. -Hold 2 – 5 breaths

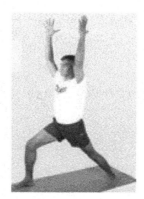

Benefits

- Chest expands

- Deep breathing

- Cures leg/neck stiffness

- Courage

Warrior-II pose

Early variation -Begin in the **warrior-I** pose.

Bend the front knee until it is directly over the ankle, make 90^0

Press the outer angle as shown; press the edge of the other foot.

Extend both arms, shoulders relaxed, twist for eyes to follow.

Hold for 3 – 5 breaths. Repeat on the other side.

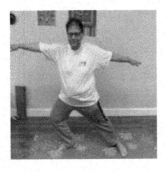 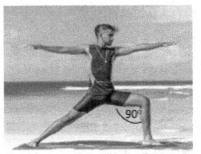

Benefits

-   Opens hips, improves balance, Strengthens shoulders, chest, and groin

Viprit Karni/Legs up the wall pose

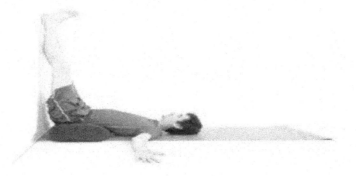

Benefits

-   Immunity/increases lymph flow

-   Soothes the heart

-   Quietens the mind

-   Calms nerves

Garudasan

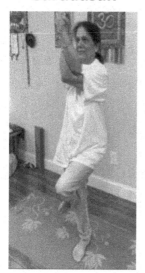

Parvatasan

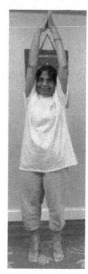

Double bind the arms and legs. Lengthen your spine, and sink deeply into your knees. Square the shoulders, keep butts and back straight.

Benefits: Stretches arms, legs

As in Tadasan,

Benefits

- Improves Balance

- Whole body-stretch

Bhujangasan

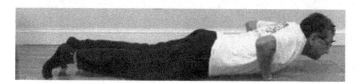

Makarasan

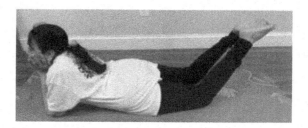

193

Naukasan

Begin in Dandasan (p.126). Bend your knees with feet flat on the floor. Raise your legs off the floor, and tilt back until you are balanced on the tail bone and two sitz bones. Inhale, and straighten your legs, creating a 30- 45-degree angle from the floor. Tighten your stomach muscles, hold 2 – 5 breaths

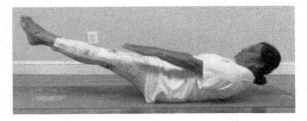

Benefits- Caution No, if having stomach pain

- Builds core muscles, heals abdominals

- Shrinks midline, prostate cure for men

- Improves stability/balance

Makarasan

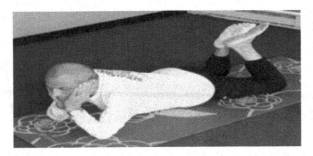

- Belly resting on the floor, legs bent toward hips

- Lie on your belly. Fold the hands to rest the chin

- Inhale, raise the chest, and the legs/Exhale to return

- Repeat 20 X

- For a more significant challenge, Join the thighs to cure high BP.

Trikonasan

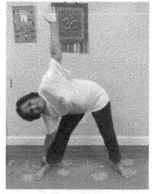
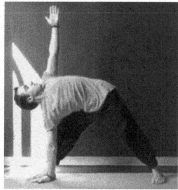

Early variation   Finish pose

Benefits-

- Relieves neck and back tension,

- Trims waist -Strengthens joints, shoulders, hips, and knees

Wind release pose (Pavan muktasan)

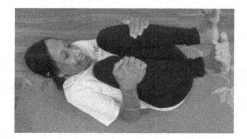

- Begin with your hips on the mat, knees drawn toward the chest, feet flexed.

- Roll your lower torso up on an exhale until your buttocks and hips are off the mat. Draw the knees toward you until your thighs rest on the chest.

- Hold for 3 – 6 breaths

Benefits

- Cures belly bloat - Backache relief

- Weight loss in the Abdomen area

PRANAYAM *P4*

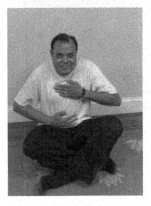
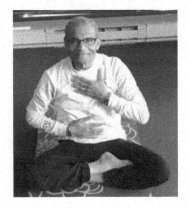

Early variation   Finish pose

Benefits

- Deep Breathing

- Focuses thought

both thighs on the ground

Hold: as long as you feel comfortable.

Ardh Matsyasan

- Sit in Lotus pose, rest elbows on the floor

- Lie on your back, holding the toes

- Inhale to gaze at the ceiling

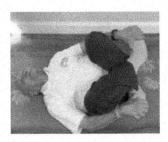

Benefits

- Stomach problems

- cures Indigestion

- Cervical pain

Utkatasan

Begin standing with your feet together; weight is on the heels. Move the hips downward. Sweep your arms front, maintaining a neutral spine.

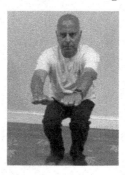

Benefits

- Strengthens thighs, upper body, & legs

- Stretches shins,

- Builds endurance

Dhanurasan

Lie full length on the floor on the stomach, face downwards. Exhale and bend the knees. Stretch arms back and hold at the ankles. Lift the head, and pull as far as possible.

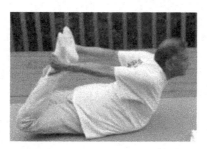

Benefits-

- Strengthens spine, shoulders, & arms

- Improves blood circulation,

- helps digestion, cures high BP

Tadasan

- Stand on both feet

- Inhale 3-sec,

- move hands up, and

- Raise both heels

Ek Padasan

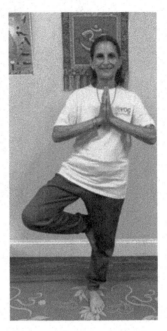

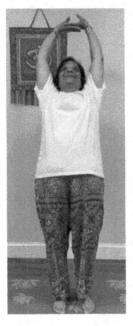

Begin standing, and transfer your weight to the left foot. Float the right foot up, and place on the left inner thigh, with your toes pointing downward. Place your hands in namaste mudra.

Benefits

- Improves Balance

- Stretches to gain height, strengthens biceps & abdominals

Benefits

- Strengthens vertebral column, inner thighs, &

- Improves balance

Shankhasan

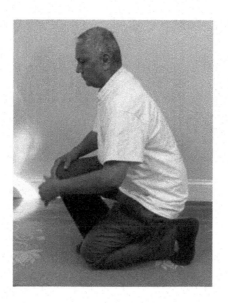

This is part of Kayakalp ayurvedic kriya

Benefits

- Obesity, diabetes

- cardio, headache

- Improves balance

- Feel light, energetic

Cow face pose

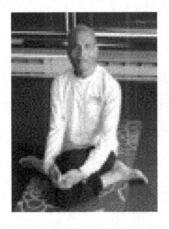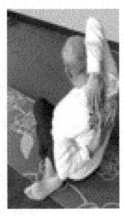

Sit tall, left knee stacked atop the other. The sit bones remain grounded. Reach your right arm, above the head, to the left arm behind. May use a towel.

Benefits

Cures cramps, improves balance, Strengthens the spine

Mandukasan

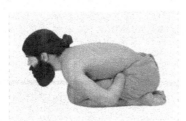

- Sit in Vajrasan pose, make a fist in both hands, and press fists on the navel.

- Exhale and bend forward for 30 sec.

- Repeat 3 X

Benefits

Cures constipation, diabetes relief

Sethubandhasan

Lying on your back, knees bent, and feet hip-width apart, engage your pelvic muscle and abdomen. Energetically draw the heel toward the head, and rise your hips.

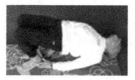

Benefits

Relieves Pain in the stomach, back, and shoulder improves immunity

Lion pose

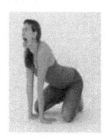

- Sit in Vajrasan pose

- Spread out knees

- fingers point back

- inhale, tongue out

- Gaze up at 3rd eye,

- Exhale and roar like a lion

- Repeat 3X

Benefits

Cures foul breath, Warms the body, Cures loss of hearing, and Speech becomes clearer

Sohum meditation

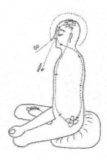

Silently, chant 'So' inhaling and 'Hum' exhaling. As you pay attention to breathing, individual & cosmic consciousness get united.

Agnisar Kriya

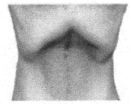

- Stand, bend at knee-hip, thighs, and torso at 90o. Start inhaling and massaging the knees.

- Now exhale completely, apply root lock, and churn the stomach rapidly for 10-20 cycles.

Benefits

Prostate care, plus constipation relief

8. MORE ASANAS FOR MINDFULNESS

Increase the duration of rechak (emptying) and kumbhak (restraining),

Konasan I: Stand erect, feet parallel 2.5 ft. apart; raise right hand to waist below ribs, the left arm on the side of thigh; turn head to look to left shoulder, inhale 3-sec bend, the right arm slides up, the left arm slides down. Come to starting position, exhaling. Repeat on the other side. 5 cycles on each side. Note the flexibility in the body.

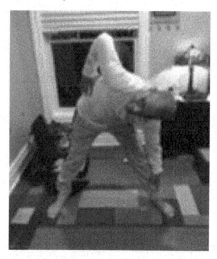

Konasana II: Stand erect, feet parallel 2.5 ft. apart; raise the right arm above the head. Head looking at a point in front, bend sideward toward the left ankle, inhaling 3s. Exhaling, return to starting position. Repeat on the other side. 5 cycles on each side.

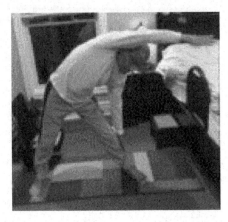

Nispand bhav: This is a technique to upgrade the power of inner hearing. Sit comfortably along the wall, spread your legs wide, and rest your hands on the thighs. Close your eyes, and pay attention to any sound coming from outside, a feeble ticking or an overhead plane roaring. Absorb in the sound; let there be no judging. Maintain the pose for 5-10 minutes. Watch that any emotion, urge, or noise is no more distracting. This is a very useful and easy kriya to let you feel relaxed instantly. **The quality and the focus change as you listen to the inner music, beyond hearing external noise.**

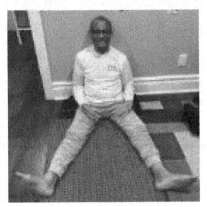

Yogmudra: Sit in Vajrasan pose and hold the right wrist in the left hand behind the back. Sit erect, and breathe normally. Bend forward, keep your neck straight, and exhale. Until your head reaches the floor, stay 30-sec max in the position.

In the next attempt, touch each knee, and stay 15 sec. Repeat each side 3X for better breathing too.

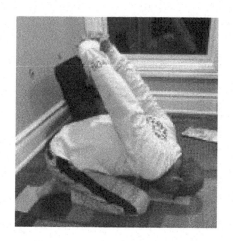

9. MYSTERY (MY STORY) OF HEALTH

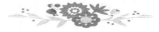

TIP 1: Good health is the sum total of good habits

TIP 2: Good habits are the outcome of Conscious living

I remember being a sickly, delicate boy in grade school, at age 13, weighing just 53 pounds.

Also, I was a shy, stuttering kid with a frail frame. My physical health improved in 2 phases

Phase I: 1954- I moved to study science in Hisar, 100 km from my hometown in Haryana. The college Principal, a father figure, took loving care of me, my diet, exercise, and study habits. I gained 10-lb in body weight and 3-inches in height in one year. My confidence grew, and I earned a better rank in the class.

Phase 2: 1959- I was earning an engineer's salary and took care of my health rationally- exploring, practicing, and adjusting my diet and walking habits, and was slowly introduced to yoga.

My health Issue	How was it improved?
i) Stutter/stammering	Practiced speaking slow with an anecdote in teaching new trainees
ii) Cold /cough/mucus flu	- Kapalbhati, lion pose, suryabhedi pranayama, - sip hot water when thirsty, - eat a spoonful of honey in ginger and black pepper daily
iii) Restless legs syndrome	March-in-place, legs up the wall, child pose and meditation at midnight

My health Issue	How was it improved?
iv) Emotional eating	Long Inhale, do Talasan/warrior pose in 3-6-3 sec
v) Drudgery / Bad mood	Bhastrika rapid breathing 15 cycles, followed by slow deep breathing
vi) Vata imbalance	Take an Ayurvedic diet (avoid cheese, dairy, stale food, eggs)/chew peppercorns. Stay warm. Meditate in Vayu mudra
vii) Constipation & high BP	
viii) Eye care	
viii) Prostate care	

TIP: Make Yog/Ayurveda/'thank you' combo an irresistible hobby of senior living.

A bonus- convert any chore, physical exercise, or walking into a conscious act [3Rs].

10. INSOMNIA: SAVASAN & YOG-NIDRA

Diet, Exercise, Sleep, Learning, & Social bonding are some of the good habits

- Sleep relaxes Brain & Meditation relaxes the Mind.

- The subtle differences between Savasan (Corpse pose) and Yog-Nidra (Guided sleep meditation) are clarified below. Pre-requisite: eat light + pranayamas*

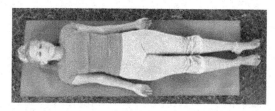

Savasan (relaxing)

Note: Savasan pose is generally practiced at the end of the yoga sequence to release tension that may have accumulated or whenever you feel fatigued. - Lie flat on your back, and keep a small folded blanket to support the curvature in the spine.

- Keep your torso/head parallel to the floor

- Be calm, with your arms resting along the sides of your body, palms facing up, eyes closed.

- Be in a relaxed, comfortable position, with tension in the back, pelvis, and legs.

- Breathe deep, equal inhale/exhale time, and observe softening of each body part one by one, from toes to the top of the head.

Yog- Nidra (guided sleep meditation)

i. Lie on your back, eyes rolled up, & feel grounded.

- Practice inhale in 2-sec/exhale in 4-sec (2 min)

ii.   Tense/Release 21 parts, one by one (2 min)

iii.   Smile & imagine your soul spirit rising out of the body, yet bonding, like a flying kite in hand

iv.   Count backward from 18 to zero, deepening the awareness of inhale/exhale-3 sec each (2 min).

v.   Scan your body from the top of the head down to the toes, experiencing relaxation growing (2 min)

vi.   Roll on your side, saying a prayer (2 min)

vii.   Continue P4 breathing, and feel a ball of white light rise till you fall asleep (total 10 min)

Insomnia: Clasp your hands tightly, interlocking the fingers. Then with left-hand fingers, press on the back of the right hand. Repeat with right-hand fingers on the back of left hand for 5 to 10 minutes in the bed.

Asanas cure: Uttanasan, Paschimottanasan, Yoni mudra & Suryabhedi pranayama without retention

11. FOUR (4) PRINCIPLES OF AYURVEDA

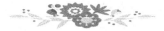

1. Introduction

- Ayurveda, the knowledge of life, is India's ancient medical system. The sister science of yoga also cures what also ails the inside body/mind through root cause analysis.

- The sage-physician Vagbhata wrote the book Ashtand Hridayam in 4th century CE, which is still used by students, teachers, physicians, and practitioners of natural cures throughout the world.

- Everyone has an innate intelligence, consisting of allotted karmas, doshas, gunas, and breaths.

It is one's duty to understand this storehouse of intelligence and keep track of how these may be upgraded/balanced in time.

2. Five (5) Elements in Ayurveda:

Human beings are made up of 5 elements

- Earth, the principle of inertia.

- Water, the principle of cohesion.

- Fire, the principle of radiance.

- Wind, the principle of vibration.

- Ether, the principle of the pervasiveness

3. Three Dosha's - *Vata – Pitta – Kapha*:

Each of us is born with a unique individual proportion of the three doshas, called our *Prakruti*. So, no two people are born alike, and more changes happen in a lifetime, which is called our *Vikruti*. When Prakruti and Vikruti numbers are understood and the balance restored, healing is faster.

Three doshas con't:

- Vata is movement

- light, dry, irregular like the air element;

- Pitta is fire and water,

- Kapha comprises Water and Earth, making Kapha the most grounded Dosha.

- My Vikruti test in 2017 showed

- Vata (12/20), Kapha (6/20), and Pitta (2/20). Vata and Kapha are, therefore, vital to my wellness. I modified what I eat and how I live to restore the digestive fire Jathragni; my mantra is Eat sattvic, well, and wise

- vegan food, and no fasting.

A Vikruti test in 2021 shows - Vata (12/20), Pitta (5/20), and Kapha (3/20). Such changes make me feel better.

4. Treatment:

My Ayurvedic awareness training in 2017 included:

- **Panchkarma:** Three basic treatments were vomiting, nasal administration, and system purification by herbs. (Laxatives or enemas are not done!)

- Suggestions for a creative routine- dincharya:

- 6 am Wake up, bowel movement, bathing,

- 8 am take b-fast, wash hands before/after eating, eat slowly, and the day spent in full awareness,

- Each day, do yogic asanas and take Ayurvedic herbs.

- Take a short walk after eating, and meditate before bedtime. Chant often, smile more often.

12. CONSTIPATION

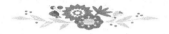

Cured the natural way- for better digestion & healthy stomach

Before - I was SAD

New habits

- No dieting or binge eating
- table sugar/refined carbs
- soft/cold/alcohol drinks
- meat, eggs, processed food
- In the morning, drink 2 c warm water, in the day 2 c herbal tea -Salty lassi at lunch, and warm water 4 c/day, dashmul Vedic powder at bedtime
- Cook vegan with extra ginger,
- whole grain roti, basmati rice

Conclusion:

In 4 months, I lost 3 kg wt & having a regular bowel movement

Now - I'm HAPPY

Asanas/Pranayamas

- AUM 3X, P1:P4, Anulom/vilom
- pawan muktasan (anti-flatus)
- Sarvangasan, Dhanurasan
- Uddiyan bandh, Kapalbhati

Shankh prakshalan poses*

- Talasan - Palm tree pose
- Tiryak Talasan
- -Swaying pose
- Kati chakrasan - waist twisting
- Tiryak bhujangasan - swaying cobra pose
- Udarakarshan - spinal twisting
- Vamandhouti (stomach wash)

Savasan, Meditation

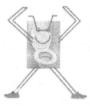

*These poses relax the muscles in the alimentary canal between stomach and anus to assist the digestive process. Lastly, treat the trip to the toilet as a purifying ritual by staying calm and waiting for spontaneous elimination. A statistic- chronic constipation has been linked to a higher risk of cardiac failure.

13. EYE CARE

Managing deadly Glaucoma with asanas and eye drops. Side benefit-improves eyesight

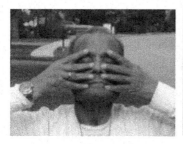
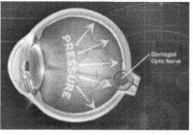

Yoni Mudra Glaucoma

Ten Remedial measures-

i) Splash cool tap water in both eyes open wide in the morning/evening or whenever needed

ii) Take Triphala powder in warm water at bedtime

iii) Sit down, and close both eyes tightly by shutting the lids. Suddenly open wide to feel the stretch. Repeat 4 times during the day.

iv) Practice Yoni mudra 2 min, followed by gently rubbing the palms and cupping the eyes. Open/close the eyes in your cupped palms 10X

v) Tratak central fixation- gaze for 1 min or more till tears flow. Mentally gaze at the third eye.

vi) Keep neck steady, look ahead, and move eyes R/L, U/D 5X, CW/CCW, 5 X

vii) Look up, move eyes half-circle, R/L, 5 X

viii) Look down, move eyes half-circle, R/L, 5 X

ix) Do modified sun salutation, chair type, 5 X

x) Acupressure treatment on eye points 4 min

What was modified

- Simplify the following Asanas in chair pose *Sarvangasan, Viprit Karni, Uttanasan*, and *Paschimottanasan* to comfort the eye, head, and heart

- Do Sitali, Nadi shodhan pranayama daily

- Computer use- Take a 20-20-20 break: every 20 minutes, deep breathe 20 seconds and look 20 feet away.

- Nasal gaze- fix the eye on the nose tip ~ 2 min.

- Adjust the chair height, and let your eyes tilt 15-deg down. Relax and pull shoulder blades down for an upright back and open chest.

CONCLUSION:

Laser surgery was postponed

I followed YOG exercises cautiously, keeping my head below the heart 15^0 or less. Fresh IOP measurement revealed a value of 12 units

14. SUN SALUTATION

SUN IS A GURU- CHANT 11 NAMES TO HONOR

1,11. Pranamasan

10.Parvatasan   2 . Parvatasa

Find an armless sturdy chair, place it on a slip-resistant yoga mat

9.Garudasan

Keep eyes closed, and hold breath to celebrate the silent …

... sensation at the end of each asana movement

3.Padhastasan

Memorize the names of asanas/mantras adds reverence to tapas

8.Pigeon pose

4.Adhomukh

7.Bhujangasan

6.Chaturangasan

5.Ekpad prasar

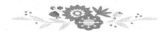

217

15. SUN SALUTATION - EXPLANATION OF BENEFITS

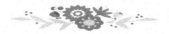

Begin with 3 rounds- gradually increase to 8 rounds in 15 minutes

Total workout for body/brain: Cardio, strength, flexibility, endurance Keep eyes open/Inhale, exhale in nose/sync mantra chanting **MANTRAS** for absorbing 11 qualities of Sun

1. Om Mitraya namah - Sun is friendly - (ॐ मित्राय नमः)

2. Om Ravayey namah - Sun is radiant - (ॐ रवये नमः)

3. Om Suryaya namah - Sun is cause of existence - (ॐ सूर्याय नमः)

4. Om Bhanavey namah - Sun illuminates the earth - (ॐ भानवे नमः)

5. Om Khagaya namah - Sun travels swiftly across the sky - (ॐ खगाय नमः)

6. Om Pusnaya namah - Sun is a star - (ॐ पूषणाय नमः)

7. Om Hiranyagarbhaya namah - Sun nourishes the world - (ॐ हिरण्यगर्भाय नमः)

8. Om Marichaya namah - Sun is Lord of dawn - (ॐ मारीचया नमः)

9. Om Adityaya namah - Sun's mom is cosmic Aditi - (ॐ आदित्याय नमः)

10. Om Bhaskaraya namah - Sun confers wisdom - (ॐ भास्कराय नमः)

11. Om Savitray namah - Sun is lord of creation - (ॐ सावित्राय नमः)

16. ASANAS ARE EXERCISES AT A SUBTLE LEVEL

Do yog to stay vibrant as you age

1. Hearing loss: Puffed cheek pose- Stand in Tadasan (mountain) pose. Eyes closed, breathe in thru both nostrils at full capacity, cheeks remaining puffed up, move chin to touch the chest. Hold till you feel pressure building up inside the ears. Move the chin up, open the eyes, and release breathing slowly thru the nose. End with a little acupressure finger.

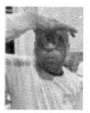

Puffed cheeks

2. Sciatica pain: Forward bend pose- Stand tall, keep feet pointing to front 2 feet apart. Bend forward over the hip joint (as shown), ensuring the back is kept flat horizontal. Place the head/hands on a chair, or use support blocks. This pose stretches the entire spine and backside, head to heels, including the hamstrings. It acts as an antidote to spine shortening caused by sitting on a desk and working.

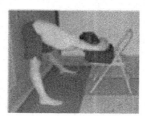

Forward bend

12. **Common cold/Flu:** Recommended asana poses are: Halasan in a chair, Viprit karni, & Savasan, including modified backbend and matsyasan for blocked nose.

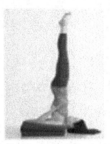

Sarvangasan

The remedy is fresh ginger pulp, ground black pepper, and honey in Ayurvedic practice. Combine the three, and gulp with warm water 3 times a day.

4. Neck pain: Stand in Tadasan pose, contracting the neck and the throat, and try to rest the chin on the chest in the notch between the collar bones and top of the breast bone.

Add Fish pose (Matsyasan) and Halasan to the usual move neck up/down front/back, CW/CCW. While the chin is pressed against the sternum. Share the bodyweight on the shoulders

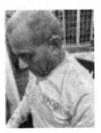

Jalandhar bandh

TIP: Art has a bad habit of prolonging, but time is limited. Exercise daily to undo stress build-up and use more time for the journey from Annamaya to pranmaya, manomay, vignanmaya kosha subtle levels of your existence

5. Strengthen Legs

5.1 Yogic walking….10 min. energizes the calf as well as thigh muscles.

5.3 In Dandasan pose, Keep palms on the thigh, heels on the ground, and flex knees 6 inches up/down. Do 50 X in 2 minutes, as rapid as possible.

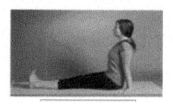

Dandasan

5.4 Raise the left leg 6 inch from the ground and hold (15 – 30 seconds). Repeat right leg.

5.5 Sit in Vajrasan, followed by Butterfly pose & Frog pose, to open the hips…2 min.

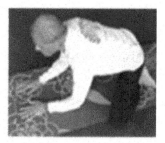

Frog pose

6. Move eyes to control the mind. Use the following guidelines

6.1 During sitting/meditating, keep the eyes closed, focusing upward to the Ajna chakra

6.2 Standing/moving in asana pose, keep eyes open to follow the hands

6.3 Ready to walk: eyes open to scan 5-10 ft ahead (inhaling) to signal safely to move.

6.4 While walking: eyes open to scan up to 50 ft inhaling, then 0-20 ft exhaling.

6.5 Sync breathing, eyes, and movements of hands and legs

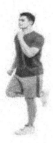

March-in-place

7. Obesity Control Recommended: Veerasan pose, Wind release pose, Boat pose, Matsyasan, Chakki chalasan, Vajrasan, Supt Vajrasan, Child pose, Cobra pose, Vakrasan, Dvichakrasan, Butterfly pose.

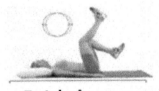

Dvichakrasan

8. Feel good anytime: Deep breathing, Brahmari pranayama, Anulom/Vilom

TIP: Rapid bhastrika pranayama promotes weight loss by inhaling oxygen O_2, and exhaling Carbon Dioxide CO_2 [inhale 32 units of O_2, exhale 44 units of CO_2, net loss 12 units/breath]

9. Memory loss is preventable: yogic wisdom: Rise from physical to mental to emotional wellness.

Mental acuity or memory loss is a major cause of worry for many seniors after reaching their 60s. This is because of their un-yogic lifestyle, engaging the senses, and not the mind and heart*

Yoga proponents claim that memory is a learned skill, "it can improve as you age" in these simple ways.

i) The mind needs variety, like the food dishes. Elevate your interest to a larger cause. Shiva(truth) and Shakti(power) reside inside you. Invite the 'Sanskrit effect' by chanting a holy mantra daily.

ii) Use the law of association, similar to a 10-digit telephone number broken into 3 chunks.

iii) Split bathing routine as steps- brushing, shampoo, massage, cupping therapy with chanting.

iv) Breathe deep often in the day- inhaling or exhaling- in awareness too.

v) Assign a spot in the house when placing the phone, wallet, or car keys.

vi) Prepare a docket that the routine stretching, twisting, and bending is now performed at a subtle level.

vii) Discover how memory notes help to improve memory?

viii) Warm-up yogic exercises: Pranayama P1.P4 & Sun salutation in chair [p.124, 125

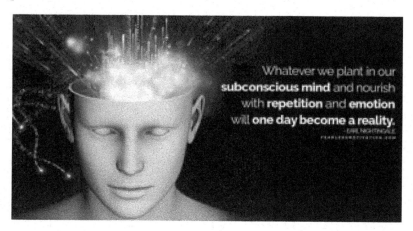

Whatever we plant in our **subconscious mind** and nourish with **repetition** and **emotion** will **one day become a reality.**

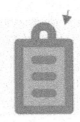

Sanskrit mantra

More yogic Asanas for enhancing memory:

- Sarvangasan (shoulder stand)

- Adhomukh (down-facing dog)

- Tadasan/Talasan (Palm tree pose)

- March-in-place (walking meditation)

- Meditation (power of silence)

* Adopt a lifestyle to elevate the total you: Body is stronger, Breathing is deeper, the lower Mind thinks better, the higher Mind inspires others too, and the spirit/Consciousness is awakening. Gradually, memory is restored, and the dependence on Rx pills also reduces.

17. YOGA FOR HIGHER VIRTUES- SIMPLIFIED

- It is human right to perform any task at a higher conscious level. Follow 3Rs: Right Intent, Right Breathing, and Right posture. Your progress is identified by Yoga becoming on-the-go joy. The first two limbs *Yamas* and *Niyamas* of Ashtang yoga may be bypassed, yet a spiritual experience right in the home setting.

- You'll observe that the physical moves/stretches can be in three distinct components:

  physical (un-conscious), mental (semi-conscious count), and Spiritual (conscious chant & count with breath on hold).

  Try to experience the higher virtue with specific asanas/kriyas, as shown below.

Asana:	Talasan	Camel pose	Cobra pose
Virtue:	Praise, worship	Humility, Confession	Physical stability

A novel yoga mat is designed with Berber carpet pieces to

i)   give acupressure treatment to hands, and feet

ii) sit, stand, lie down safely without slipping

iii) enhancing the higher feel

iv) regulate physical moves in narrow limits, and you're

v)   enhancing the superior feel faster than before.

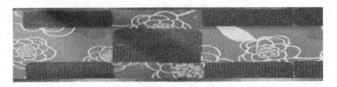

Novel Yoga Mat

18. NOVEL WELLNESS REPORT

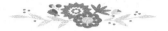

12 new tests: to know yourself better [1]

1. Body Mass Index (BMI)......Your height/waist ratio (healthy body > 2)

2. Chest expansion on inhaling .... 2% or more healthy (1% or less unhealthy)

3. Resting heart rate.... (60-80 BPM healthy/>100 sign of sickness)

4. Breathing ... avoid shallow breathing unconsciously by the mouth

   Make deep breathing 12-15 bpm by the nose (a conscious habit for better health)

5. Toilet habit... daily bowel moving-healthy/irregular - sickness

6. Sleep quality... 7-8 hours healthy/insomnia – impending sickness

7. Bone mineral density test (DXA scan)- as advised by your physician

8. Purity practice.... Cleansing/detoxing by daily, weekly, monthly, annual routine ...

9. Doshas ...Know your Ayurvedic humor Vata, Pita, Kapha, to adjust your diet/supplements

10. Gunas (sattva, rajas or tamas). To learn the art of balancing.

11. Time/Energy allocation ...to physical, mental, emotional, and meditative activities

12. Health Journal ... Record preventive measures: diagnostic tests, vaccine shots, asana poses

---

(1) The usual Five (5) screening tests for seniors are- Blood pressure, glucose, Cholesterol, Colorectal Cancer, and Prostate cancer. To evaluate Total health, 12 new tests are proposed.

(2) Ex. To lose 2-pounds, cut your diet by 7 000 calories; hence the better option is yog + diet

(3) You begin to self-diagnose/live a lifestyle to suit your health category.

TIP: In my case- I avoided cheese, corn, dairy milk, eggs, non-veg, stale, or left-over CRAP food.

Also, I discovered the power of the mind at the time of meditation-sadhana. If I focused on what is good in my life, I would create more of it. Also, appreciate why I am unique individually yet familiar at a cosmic level.

TIP: Life must be lived forward but can only be understood backward.

19. NOVEL GREETING CARD DESIGN

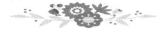

Yoga dances and games are well-known entertainment themes. The novel theme is to make a yogic Greeting card. More people doing Yoga now means more healthy individuals, lower cost of health insurance, and direct savings to Medicare, leaving guaranteed monetary benefits to the future generation.

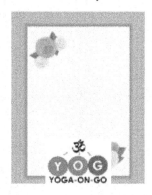

May Yog craft your destiny

Do Yog together to take better care of both

May you thrive like a lotus flower: be in the world but not of it

Celebrate Ekadashi day with the Yagna havan ritual,

to create the right environment

May a thing larger than memory manifest your life

May you discover that Science & Spirituality are not at loggerheads

May you practice pranayamas & Suryanamaskar daily

May 3Rs guide your actions, thoughts, and emotion

Make Yog a new mantra for peace of mind, health, prosperity, and wow!

May your bond with yourself and others strengthen by Namaste & AUM chanting

May you meditate daily for 10 minutes in the morning and evening

May you proudly say, 'I do, Yog, why don't you.'

May you discover that the sweetest person on earth is in the mirror

Begin the day smiling right in the bed

19. NOVEL GREETING CARD DESIGN

Enjoy your big day in the novel yogic way

To love spouse is karma, love each other is dharma

20. CONCLUSION: PART THREE

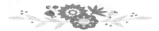

- **The project of writing** the eBook has been a thrilling 4-stage experience. i) Tadbhuddhaya ii) tadatmanah iii) tannishtha iv) tadparaynah.

  i) learn, ii) understand, iii) analyze, and iv) transfer the knowledge to others

  Absorb in your mind, be passionate, self-experience, and inspire others

- **Struggles and problems** are part of life, but stress/anxiety are artificial.

- Analyze pain, or discomfort for learning a new lesson, or the 3-stage growth

- **Intelligent/un-selfish:** You can transform into an intelligent, un-selfish being.

  Then your 'real' selfless identity follows, like a divine consort.

- **Say no to fault-finding.** Not your business to point the finger at another person as 3 fingers point back at you. However, feel free to compliment and win 3X praise in return. 300% ROI. Wow!

Pointing finger

- **Say yes to Yog.** Emotional distress or boredom is an opportunity to step up the yoga effort, get healed without drinking alcohol, and earn merit.

- **Purity practice:** A side benefit is Purity practice in all realms. I started saying 'No' to added sugar and added daily meditation to my routine.

  If the action was not taken at a younger age, it takes more effort to outdo a bad habit.

- **A yogi** wisely enjoys dual citizenship- initially the outer physical world of Body/Mind. Later, he consciously studies yoga before retiring into his golden years of life.

Prayer nook

TIP: Sit in silence at the prayer-cum-yoga-nook in every home, school, or hospital.

Lessons learned while writing the Book..........

1. Challenge your knowledge in the following areas

    -   Risk of carrying (i) extra body weight and (ii) past grievances

    -   Risk of not knowing what is a preventable or treatable illness

    -   Risk of staying home, separation, no church-going, vanishing faith or cultural traditions

    -   Risk of over-eating, wasting food, time, and resources, even if you can afford financially

    -   Risk of developing chronic sickness, and aging/dying prematurely

2. By doing daily Yog, one can utilize the wired intelligence to stay ever exuberant, and

    -   to Spend the aloneness on healthy positive thinking, and better body behavior

    -   to say No to depression, despair, and fear, express gratitude to the caregiver (why suffer in silence?)

    -   to spread the message that in times of sickness, our organs heal better and faster, as warmth is shared without resistance as you are less worried

3. Ahamkar, the fake ego of I, me, mine, is the biggest obstacle in the spiritual journey. Its antidote is positive svabhiman- Amness resulting in

ripple-free Consciousness. YOG teaches - how best to balance the two opposites?

'Namo Arihantanam' – is a prayer on the same theme by the Jainas

'Ek Omkar Sat Nam...gurprasad' The One Reality is known by Guru's grace- is a prayer in the Sikh faith.

Make these or similar mantras part of daily practice to awaken the Amness

4. End Prayer: 'Sarve bhavantu sukhina .....Aum Shantih' is an old-time Hindu prayer!

May the goodwill and yogic transformation touch many hearts and minds

ACKNOWLEDGMENTS

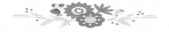

First, thanks to my loving wife, (late) Vinod Rustagi. Her life has been a continuing inspiration- how to be healthy till the final breath? That meant that a retiree's life has not to end in fighting illnesses, taking pills and more pills, or dying in a hospice or long-term care home. Instead, Yoga, and more yoga, live healthily, then pass quietly, chanting the Mahamrityunjay mantra, a song of victory over death.

Thank you to my elder son Rajat Rustagi, and his wife Anju, to my younger son Saras Rustagi and his

wife, Nitu. The greatest reward is the keen interest of my grandkids, Rohit, Rea, and Rayna - their significant achievements in school and college are already bringing glory to the Rustagi family in America. In them, I regularly see a glimpse of living divinity. Their collective caring in my advanced age has encouraged the yoga Book.

To my brother Dharam Vir and sister, Pushpa, residing in India, their fathomless love lets me thrive through YOG practice and writing.

The New York Sports Club (NYSC), where I witness young adults and seniors working out and in love with their bodies. What I like most in the Gym is setting a new healthy America on the horizon.

Health and education, family, and yoga would ultimately link all the more than seven billion people globally. These are the interesting topics everyone likes to talk about or brag about, which added value to my office work trips worldwide.

To my role models - Dr. Navneet Arora, professor of Engineering at IIT Roorkee, India, and to Mr. Vishwambhar 'Vishu' Sharma, a reputed author on spiritual books, de-coding the Upanishadic wisdom.

Thanks to Ms. Deepti Rastogi, she promptly designed the colorful Logo: Yoga-On-Go.

To Ms. Rea Rustagi, a math student at Columbia University, for making quality sketches, and 12 y/o Rayna Rustagi for posing for yoga pics.

I humbly acknowledge the contributions of the members of the Sambandh yoga group for their dedication to practicing Asanas, especially to Daksha & Hemendra Patel for generously allowing the use of their home for Monday classes. Kulin Hemani, Kirit Kothari, Ashwin Parikh, & Dr. Satish Mullick deserve special mention for their constant encouragement and organizing the promotional events.

Regards and thanks to Tarun Mehta, Jayu Parikh, Deepak Sethi, and Surendra Jain for holding yoga classes during the current pandemic, and to Surekha Khedekar for amazing photographs in the Book.

Also, to my first client Kathleen Bedoya for believing that YOG and meditation would help her son get better grades in the Montclair high school.

I am ever grateful to my alma-mater 'The Yoga Institute' in Mumbai, India, for accepting me as a student in their 200-hour Teacher Training program in March 2015. Madam Hansaji Yogendra, the distinguished Director of TYI, shared the vision that learning is not limited by chronological age.

To Prof. Dr. K Muraleedharan Nair, Director of Vaidyaratnam Ayurveda Foundation in Thrissur, Kerala, India, an author, encouraged me to write the e-book.

Thanks to pixabay.com, unsplash.com, freeart.com, and royalty-free.com for using their images.

Amit P Sharma's professional editing effort in getting the book in its current format is acknowledged.

Lastly, thanks to the Sambandh EC board- Nitin Maniar, Urvashi & Veral Patel, Neeta Juvekar, Dr. Pradip Shah, and Anurag Rochlani for their positive feedback on the activities of the vibrant Yoga group.

ABOUT THE AUTHOR

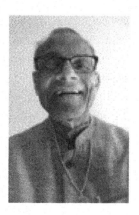

Prof. Raghuvir 'Ravi' Rustagi is 86 y/o

- a professional engineer, yoga instructor, an author, and a volunteer

- born in East Panjab in the time of the British raj- now Haryana, India

- studied at Delhi college of engineering, IIT Mumbai, and ORNL, Tenn. USA

- a designer/inventor with professional experience in India & America

- travelled to many countries where commercial nuclear power plants operate

- currently living in NJ, USA, embracing his Indian background in the U.S. setting

- a licensed yoga teacher with a passion for combining yoga, meditation, and modern technology to spread health awareness; he relishes proving yogic benefits to himself.

- in pandemic times, teaches zoom class every Monday voluntarily

- he applied the logic of nuclear data and analysis to conclude that yogic intervention can be an added weapon to fight all strains of COVID-19.

- he believes that a yogi derives natural protection from infections and chronic illnesses through disciplined living, early detection, prevention, and treatment regardless of age.

Getting personal- A nuclear scientist and a religionist. I don't drink, don't smoke, take no Rx, do no drugs. I cook and eat a vegan, egg-free meal, do yoga and meditate. Trust in one God- manifesting all beings and things- has guided my life and career decisions throughout. When I take time to read religious scriptures, Bhagavad Gita, Ramayana, or Yog-sutra, and pray in the Hindu faith, it makes me feel fitter in body and calm in mind. The energy in the distant Sun is nuclear fusion, and ultimately man must design safer and better fusion-based nuclear plants on earth.

Till then, melt-free nuclear fission reactors need to be built, such as SMR (small modular reactor)

In 2005, Prof. Rustagi formally retired from the nuclear profession and settled in the scenic hills of Schuylkill County, Pennsylvania. The Pennsylvania State University's local campus offered him to teach four undergraduate courses in Engineering Mechanics and College Algebra as an Adjunct Professor. This was an opportunity to interact with young, responsible adults. Prof Rustagi introduced deep breathing in the classroom to gain students' focus on solving STEM (science, technology, engineering & mathematics) problems.

In 2015, a pursuit began in the area of health and wellness through Yoga & Ayurveda. He obtained a 200-hour Teacher Training license from the world fame, 'The Yoga Institute' in Santa Cruz East, Mumbai, India. He also completed an Ayurveda Awareness course in 2017 at 'The Vaidyaratnam Ayurvedic Foundation' in Thrissur, Kerala. According to what a senior may safely accomplish, he learned to modify or use supports to simplify the complex Asana poses. He usually verifies the benefit of a posture beforehand, and his teaching style continues to appeal to young adults and seniors. He coined a new term YOG 'Yoga-On-Go' -both noun and verb to promote a yogic lifestyle of choice.

Yoga of mindfulness syncing the physical, emotional, and spiritual bodies is a total experience and can be within reach of all people. Just follow 3Rs.

The eBook 'yoga on go' has grown from handouts to students of Sambandh Yoga Group, a Sanskriti of NJ initiative www.sanskritiofnj.org.

Prof. Rustagi lives in Livingston, NJ, USA, and in Dwarka, New Delhi, when in India.

Sincere regards to Ms. Falguni Pandya, IYD Event Chair for inspiring residents of Livingston NJ

REFERENCES

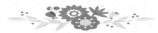

1. Iyengar, BKS. Light on Yoga. :Schocken Books, Inc.: New York, NY, 1979

2. Lad, Vasant Dr. Ayurveda- a practical guide. Lotus press.: Twin Lakes, WI, USA, 2009

3. Yogendra, Jaydeva Dr. Cyclopedia Yoga. :The Yoga Institute, Santa Cruz(East): Mumbai- 400055, India, 2015

4. Ramdev, Swami. YOG Sadhna.: Diamond Pocket books (pvt) Ltd.:Faridabad, India 110022

5. Rajendra Atal, Acharya. :YOG evam Prakrutik Chikitsa: Suruchi Prakashan, New Delhi-11055, 2017

6. Vohra, Devendra. Health in your Hands: Navneet Publications (I) Ltd, Mumbai, India, 1998

7. Rustagi, Ravi. : Havan Ritual Made Easy: www.Google.com, USA, 2022